TIMELESS

TIMELESS

*The Journey to Discover
Life's Greatest Secret*

KATHY BROOK &
VICTOR BROOK

NEW YORK

LONDON • NASHVILLE • MELBOURNE • VANCOUVER

TIMELESS
The Journey to Discover Life's Greatest Secret

Published in New York, New York, by Morgan James Publishing. Morgan James is a trademark of Morgan James, LLC. www.MorganJamesPublishing.com

Scripture quotations marked (NIV) are taken from the Holy Bible, New International Version®, NIV®. Copyright © 1973, 1978, 1984, 2011 by Biblica, Inc.™ Used by permission of Zondervan. All rights reserved worldwide. www.zondervan.comThe "NIV" and "New International Version" are trademarks registered in the United States Patent and Trademark Office by Biblica, Inc.™

Morgan James BOGO™

A **FREE** ebook edition is available for you or a friend with the purchase of this print book.

CLEARLY SIGN YOUR NAME ABOVE

Instructions to claim your free ebook edition:
1. Visit MorganJamesBOGO.com
2. Sign your name CLEARLY in the space above
3. Complete the form and submit a photo of this entire page
4. You or your friend can download the ebook to your preferred device

ISBN 978-1-63195-369-9 paperback
ISBN 978-1-63195-370-5 eBook
Library of Congress Control Number: 2020920345

Cover Design by:
Rachel Lopez
www.r2cdesign.com

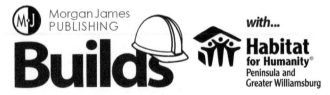

Morgan James is a proud partner of Habitat for Humanity Peninsula and Greater Williamsburg. Partners in building since 2006.

Get involved today! Visit
MorganJamesPublishing.com/giving-back

With all of our hearts we dedicate
this journey to our four children,
Hunter, Audrey, Olivia, and Averie,
who have inspired, challenged, and
walked with us with Love, Faith and Grace.

TABLE OF CONTENTS

FOREWORD

When I heard that my dear friends, Kathy and Victor were embarking on a new adventure writing *Timeless*, I couldn't have been more excited and happy to watch this culmination of information come into existence. How refreshing to take real life experience and fiction and put them together for an amazing journey to find out what life's greatest secret is…a different experience for every reader. In all of my years, I have learned that we are all on different paths and that there are so many forks in the road where we must choose our direction. *Timeless* lets your imagination run free so you can take your own individual path and see where you go.

I've known Kathy and Victor since their children were in grade school. I watched this couple running the roads, dropping kids of at soccer, track & field and gymnastics practices, etc., attending every single academic, social, or athletic event. What a pace! I am always interested in how people tick and would frequently ask how they were doing. I would always get the same answer: "It's all great, everything is going great." I believe the only way they could possibly have handled this machine of a family was to keep their heads up and move forward with this positive attitude. As a former college basketball player, air force officer, business owner and entrepreneur, husband, father and grandfather, I live life with the same philosophy, to be a man who always keeps up the pace using positivity. I understand having lots of moving parts, and the importance of lifting up others, making people feel as important as they truly are. This is the essence of Kathy and Victor and the dynamic energy they share.

Kathy was the fitness trainer to the love of my life and wife, Mary. I would go with Mary on occasion to walk on the treadmill during her sessions. Kathy, a woman with a beautiful smile, would ask questions about my health and exercise routine. We spoke about weekly golf outings with close buddies and my college career as an SMU Mustang basketball player, when we won two Southwest Conference championships (1955 & 1956) and even made it to the NCAA Final Four my senior year, and I would explain that weights and machines were not a priority back in the day. She introduced different routines and before I knew it, her confidence had me hooked, and I was soon working out with her as well. Kathy reminded me of a young female version of myself, energetic with a desire to help others is just in our blood. I knew the protocol and welcomed it happily.

Victor, being disciplined in his personal life as well as his own workout regimens, would occasionally be at the gym at the same time. We shared many conversations about life, family, and the art of getting young athletes into these top tier universities. I grew to understand the time and commitment associated with this process, and was very intrigued to say the least.

Over the years, a beautiful bond between the four of us grew. We were no longer just friendly acquaintances twice a week. We shared many victories and losses, and it just felt like family.

It is with loving gratitude that I look forward to being a part of their journey and watching them achieve this dream. And I'm thrilled that you get to come along as well.

Tom Miller

President, Aucoin & Miller Electrical Supply Company

AUTHOR'S NOTE

This story you are about to read is an allegorical journey in which a traveler sets out on an expedition to discover life's greatest secret . . .

What is time?
How is it measured?
Can we affect time?
How can it be optimized to fulfill life's perfect line?

Here we've blended elements of reality, fantasy, history, spirituality, and science to cover the four corners of the earth—the narrator armed with an unquenchable thirst for destiny's call to understand the truth of human experience. Watch the narrator discover artifacts and allow them to guide his journey with lessons from ancient civilizations.

You, too, just might . . . cascade through time.

Prologue

DISCOVERY VOYAGE

It's the beginning of a new time for me.

I've been waiting for this day for a long time . . . years, in fact.

I'm excited, yet calm. This date has been circled on my calendar for some time, and I've been counting down the days. For so long, it was just this date in the future, but as it came within reach, I started believing that it could become reality. It could actually be real.

The car is picking me up in a few hours to take me to the airport for this long-awaited, dreamed-of experience. It will hopefully be the start of a new day, a new life, a new time for me. I've spent years getting to this point . . . So much hard work has gone into arriving at this special day. All the research and interviews, the dead ends, starting over, again, and again, and again. The rabbit trails leading to another fork in the road, another wrong turn, scrapped plans, crumpled up paper over by the trash can, and back to the drawing board once more.

Many times, I felt like it couldn't happen. I would pause to look over my shoulder, checking whether anyone was watching me go just a little crazy in the pursuit of something that might not even be based in reality.

What was I doing anyway?

What made me think that I possessed any unique gifts or skills that would grant me access to one of life's most sought-after treasures?

Yeah, I had a lot of life experience, as well as significant training in academia and research. I had degrees from universities, elite institutions that gave me impressive pieces of sheepskin to display on my wall. I had certainly seen a few things in life over the years, but I think that's pretty normal. I figure most people on this planet have had similar life experiences as me. There's nothing special there.

I do, however, possess a dogged, thick skin, a never-quit mentality that I cling to every day. (Okay, some might call it a chip on my shoulder.) I would find it, or I would spend all of my days fighting toward that end. It was that important. It mattered that much—or at least it did to me. It partly mattered because I wanted the world to know that my heart was full. I was destined to reach this place, this standing in life. But I also knew its value in the quiet moments, when I was almost daydreaming, looking across the room or staring at the stars, wondering: What am I doing here? What is my purpose? Is there really a plan for me, or is that just for those other people, the ones I've always heard and read about becoming successful or accomplished, inventing something, or just simply being famous for one reason or another?

I guess, somewhere along the way, I started to adopt my plan, to take some ownership of it—or, at least, privately I did. I didn't really tell anyone what I was thinking, or what I was trying to do, or what research I was undertaking. I don't know why. Maybe it's that little voice that makes us keep things to ourselves out of fear that someone will shoot down our dreams, our thoughts, our ideas. Finally, I reached the point when I started to really believe in this wild concept, this amazing path that I would follow. Where would it take me? That eventually became a driving force for me and, ultimately, a lot of the fun. Like a secret only I possessed.

I wasn't completely sure, of course. It's kind of like playing that game where you surprise someone by taking out a map, having them close their eyes, turning them around, and then just pointing to a spot on the map to head off on a journey that doesn't have a known end. What are the stops that you will take along the way, the experiences you will have, or the people you will meet? It doesn't matter. You just go. In fact, I started living by this daily saying:

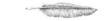

Trust in God and take another step.

It became my mantra, calming me and giving me strength.

Then, one day, I just knew. I really knew. I knew completely that it was, in fact, real. I hadn't seen it yet, but I just knew. It was real. And this was my destiny. I had been planning for this my whole life.

It would be wonderful to have known ahead of time or to have some element of confidence for the greater part of my life that this was my life plan, but that's just not how it works for most people, and it was no different for me. I could have used a special guide, an angel taking me this way and that rather than not knowing why I had to go through all of the stuff throughout my life—but now I know. That stuff helped me develop my thick skin and the survival instincts to ultimately reach my destination. To be able to arrive at this very point in time, when I would finally take this ultimate journey for which my entire life has been prepping me.

Once I knew, really knew, I finally started sharing my vision with my very closest confidant. I opened up a little, took some risks to express what I was thinking, laid out my actual plans. It felt like a vulnerability to open up like that; yet, it offered an opportunity to relieve what had been banging around in only my head for so long. I could finally ask someone to accept my point of view and maybe even embrace it.

My confidant's response wasn't the one I was expecting, although I'm not sure what response I was hoping for, or if I had even really thought about it. But she did receive what I shared with love and the intention to try to grasp why it took me some time to work up the nerve to say what I did.

Honestly, what else could I expect? Relative to the norms, my ideas were a little ways from having both feet firmly on the ground. They were certainly removed from traditional thoughts of gravity.

Thankfully, however, that was it, the day I knew for certain, the beginning of the fulfillment of what was to come. Maybe it was because I spoke the words out loud or told another soul, or maybe it was just that nothing spectacularly awful happened to me after vocalizing the words. Whatever the reason, it became illuminatingly clear that it didn't matter how long it took or what obstacles there were during the challenging road ahead. If someone laughed at me or mocked my daily activities, it just didn't seem to matter anymore. It was like having a secret that only I knew. A superior sense of strength came from knowing both the secret and the goal. I didn't create it, mind you. I was just going to unlock it, be the torchbearer, and ultimately share it with the world. This wasn't for someone to keep under lock and key in a safe or mountain hideaway. It was bigger than that. It was the search of a lifetime meant to be available to everyone.

My drive really picked up at that point. I wanted it more than you could imagine. Have you ever had one of those experiences where you just couldn't sleep you were so driven? Something drove your every thought? You go to bed at night thinking about it and you are already thinking about brewing your coffee early in the morning (yes, actually smelling the aroma and tasting it) in order to get started on the project again the next day?

Then it happened. Everything began to fall into place. Like one of those once-in-a-lifetime stories about the planets aligning. They weren't aligned yet, but you could certainly tell, without a doubt, it was happening. One of the planets is a little to the left and too high and another too far to the right, but it is conceivable that they could eventually come together.

That day was it for me.

The planets were beginning to align. I had certainly not arrived; however, I was on the path toward arrival, and I knew it.

One discovery led to another and another and another. The real test would be whether the discoveries started canceling each other out, or whether they would continue to make sense and support the position I had been formulating. All of these clues and seemingly unconnected pieces of information . . . In some cases, they didn't make sense at all, but I just kept believing. I'm not sure why . . . Some childlike faith, I guess. Or maybe just blind hope.

By that stage in my search, even if it didn't exist, I didn't care. The passion I felt doing what I loved was worth spending all of my days and nights, for that matter forever, in the pursuit of a dream. It reached the point that, even if it wasn't real, I would rather believe it was than live without the hunger and passion that this pursuit had given me each day.

You see, I'm one of those people who doesn't need to see something to get excited about it. Imagining the possibilities is the greatest exhilaration of all—and most of the fun.

Don't get me wrong now, I'm beyond thrilled that it exists and that I'm on the last leg of this journey to uncover its riches. But, if it weren't, I've received so much joy in the years I've spent pursuing this destiny that I feel accomplished and blessed to have lived such a fascinating and full existence by this stage in my life.

Besides, with all of my notes and directions, along with the guidance of the many amazing, talented specialists who've offered their expertise along the way, if it were not me, someone else with diligent commitment would have come to these conclusions and located it sooner or later.

But it's almost time now.

As I look around my library, I see all the memories, everything that has brought me to this point.

There are so many books, notes, scratch pads, maps, and tools of the trade. It's a little messy, but there's still some sort of strange organization to it all. Over in the corner of my credenza is a stack of all my travel itineraries, plane tickets, hotel reservations, rental car receipts, and cards from my interesting restaurant choices during my glorious travels all over the world. Like the one in Marrakech that offered those famous tagines, a delectable stew prepared in a shallow, circular clay cooking pot by the same name, Arabian spices, Spanish olive oils, slow-cooked lamb with honey-soaked prunes and crunchy fried almonds, or phyllo pastry stuffed with chicken, onions, eggs, sugar, and ground almonds, all orchestrated by the Jewish Moors preservation techniques. Or like the French protectorate cafe styles creating an intersection of culinary delights, served with preserved lemons and smen. It's not the faint traveler who finds the traditional local Moroccan cafes, likely a converted residence, as the corridors twist and turn around the Medina markets, where the streets are lined with vendors and shop owners promoting their wares. I'm usually able to find an idyllic second story outdoor ledge cafe spot to sip mint tea as the sun sets and late afternoon festivities take place below. The aroma and flavor of the specialty mint tea alone is worth the trip.

For a moment, I just stare with a real sense of accomplishment at the memories. With a slight grin out of the left corner of my mouth,

I reflect on all the time I've put in to get to this point. The passion that drove me, day after day, never letting me down. For sure, there were some really hard days. Days when I felt like I would never get there or that it was just a hopeless dream, a fantasy. Days when I felt it wasn't real or experienced the looming question: Is this really worth it?

But, thankfully, something kept me going.

Something inside me kept lifting and driving me to get up and go again, to just take one more step. To drive forward and keep believing that all of my life's work would culminate in this very day. That I would eventually arrive at the special place that was shouting my name.

Well, that day has finally arrived. It's been circled on the calendar and come to fruition. I'm truly going on the trip of a lifetime.

Looking back, it's a little surreal because it shouldn't have taken me this long to get here. I just kept missing all of the signs. I kept thinking that it can't possibly be this simple. And why shouldn't I think that? Men and women much better than me have searched forever, yet still come up short. So why would I be able to make this discovery? It just couldn't be this simple. It was right under my nose the whole time, and I just couldn't see it—or just couldn't accept it.

I shouldn't be so hard on myself, I suppose. It's all I knew. All my training was wrong. The things I've always thought were right were sometimes a little bit of a miss or off just enough that, of course, I would angle off one way or the other, or go down the wrong trail by a degree here and there, and end up following the wrong path.

The amazing thing is, the right path was trying so hard to present itself, but, as I eventually learned, there was a significant amount of fine-tuning that needed to be dialed in (or practiced more frequently) for it to become second nature. The right path isn't an expression of my academic acumen, my distinctive training as a historian or philosopher (although I'm truly an explorer at heart), the degrees or the institutions

I've attended, the parchments hanging in my study . . . it's more of an intuition, an understanding of life that comes from somewhere else, an internal guide, or even a higher power, perhaps.

There is some real satisfaction though because something tells me that if I had not had to go through all that I did, it may not be as precious. It might not mean as much to me as it does now if I'd seen the right path from the get-go. So, all I feel at this point is gratitude, a sense of accomplishment, and appreciation for this journey.

Okay, it really is time for me to get ready to go. All my clothes are laid out on the bed. Up until now, they have been hanging on the right side of the closet in anticipation of the day when I would reach up and grab them to go on this special trip. It's all here: my Indiana Jones look-alike outfit, the shirt and pants and, of course, that hat, plus all the critical tools of the trade, including compass, maps, notebook, shoulder satchel . . . and bullwhip.

The whip simply became a sort of enjoyable sidearm, if you will, to get me in the spirit over the years during all of my research. I would hold it and act out the snap of the whip just to create a focused mood and return to the goal at hand. Similar to how listening to a certain song puts you in a specific place and time almost instantly, the whip reminded me why I was here and of my true purpose. I would grab the whip, smell the leather, unwrap it to full length, twirl it around a little, then snap it across the library toward an old collector's saddle that I picked up years ago, trying to hit the saddle horn. I actually got pretty good at it as this became my preparation for clear thinking, a lamp-light-goes-on ritual.

Ah, I hear the car. It has just pulled up to the curb to pick me up and head to the airport hangar where the plane sits, flight plan already approved, completely fueled and ready to go.

When we arrive at the hangar, I step out of the car and thank the driver. Everything seems so surreal. Am I in a movie theater, watching the release of that new blockbuster action film that the whole world has been anticipating—or is this actual life? Ouch, that hurt! I slam my head against a lower corner of the ceiling as I step down to the stairs toward the level where the plane rests. Yes, this is real. Let's not do that again.

I board the passenger section of a twin-engine aircraft. It looks just like many that I have hopped aboard before, ones that look like they may or may not be able to actually complete the mission. I can smell that distinctive leather that only comes from a small aircraft like this one. I duck my head through the tiny entry and climb aboard. No one else is here, except for the pilot. I can see his right shoulder and arm fiddling with the dials, conducting some mumbling sounds (to the tower, I presume). Otherwise, it's empty. I guess it would be. Who am I expecting anyway? This is a journey that I have always trekked on my own, and now it's obvious why. I suppose we all must forge our own way. Storing my backpack and satchel under the seat in front of me, I begin to sweat from the tiny cabin. Of course, the air conditioning is not on yet.

The pilot hits the ignition and the engines slowly start grinding. The left one engages, then the right. That familiar vibration is in full swing as the entire plane begins to shimmy and hum. This is really happening. The anticipation is mounting. I'm literally like a little kid at an amusement park. I remember those days, standing in line with my family and friends when I was a child. The lines didn't seem long then. It was too exciting to be a chore. That childlike feeling of 'I can do anything,' no dream or mission is too big. Every time we would turn another corner, I could see a different angle of the boxcar train streaming along the tracks. The back, then the side or underneath as it thundered around the bend. Every time it came around, I would get up on my tippy toes and reach my neck as far as I could to see through that little gap between the tracks and the enormous steel frame holding them up. It gets louder and louder. Then I see that red train coaster streaming away from me on those round blue curling pipes that seem like they could hold up a rocket ship.

It's that same wonder and excitement that grip me as we begin to taxi out to the runway. I can barely see the pilot with his headset, but I can tell that he is saying something. I'm assuming he's getting permission from the air traffic controllers to take off and asking for any final instructions to the cockpit.

All of the sudden, the roar of the engines starts to increase, and the noise grows as we began to move. At least, I think we are moving. Yes, we are definitely moving and shaking and rattling down the runway we go. My head feels glued back against the headrest as I lie back in my seat.

In an instant, we are weightless and lifting away from the earth. I turn to the left, looking out the not-made-for-looking-out window as we rise and gain distance from the ground below. I've flown many times before, but I'm still amazed by the ability of humans to fly through the air, no matter the mode.

Airborne, and aware that we have a long way to go, I ponder what to do with my time. Reaching for my black, soft leather briefcase, feeling that I should be doing something, I start reviewing all of my notes, painstakingly outlined, with every detail pinpointed.

As I do so, I realize that I'm ready. It's already done. The work has been completed, almost to the point of excess. The hay is in the barn, as they say.

Of course, it should be, I've been preparing for so long and I've had plenty of time to make sure that this one most important trip of a lifetime was going to go off without a hitch. It was going to bear fruit and produce the results I have dreamed about for most of my life. With the constant buzzing of the engines and the surprisingly comfortable seat, I nodded off for what seemed to be just a couple of minutes.

A big bump awakes me, and I hear the sound of the landing gear being deployed while the descent is already underway. We must be close. As I look out the window, I see nothing but water. I rub my eyes and crane my neck to look through the tiny window, finally seeing the shore. There, in the very bottom corner edge of the window, I can see land. It continues to grow, and eventually the landing strip exposes itself, just beyond the beach. Nothing sophisticated. Just a simple dirt track cut through the jungle. Created for the single purpose of landing small planes on this remote destination. Long enough, I suspect, to land our small craft safely and secure—at least, I hope.

The pilot descends rapidly, causing vibrations and rattling again from the seat I'm strapped into as we decline beneath the tree line. The rear wheels of the plane settle on the dirt track, followed by the front one. The brakes and wing levers, fully engaged now, easily press my head forward as we begin to slow, and comfort starts to take center stage as it's now obvious that we are going to survive, come to a complete stop, and be able to live another day.

Once the plane comes to a stop and the pilot shuts down the engines, a small light comes through the door. I peek my head around the corner to see a single man standing and waiting. I begin to deplane once given clearance by the pilot, descending down the manually attached ladder. Seemingly a local, with a big smile on his face, he says with a heavy accent something creatively interpreted by me to mean, "Welcome to my island! How was your trip?"

Somewhat blinded by the light and trying to make him out clearly, I say thank you.

We open the luggage hatch and grab the few belongings needed for our long expedition ahead. With several hours of daylight still available, we load up and march ahead.

My guide is very simply dressed in an old, tan, slightly torn shirt made from some type of animal skin, baggy potato-sack pants with a drawstring around the waist, and a pair of homemade sandals. He is carrying a huge machete in his right hand with a slight grin—at least, I think it's a grin—on his face. He speaks a sort of broken English, but it's enough for us to communicate effectively. Between his hand motions and me picking up a word here and there, I gather that he is asking me to follow him, so I do as instructed.

Just a few steps into our trek, we are surrounded by a complete blanket of green landscape, quickly consumed by the jungle. Vines and heavy wild foliage cover the earth in every direction as far as the eye can see, which is somewhat limited due to the thickness of the landscape. Hence, the machete, and the know-how to use it, is immediately on display.

We begin what I expected to be a several-day journey through unforgiving terrain. The temperature is nice, pleasant in fact. Not at all what I expected. There's even a cool, light breeze that shows itself every few seconds, making the experience much more pleasant.

We walk, eat, camp, light a fire, and get a few hours of rest each night. Morning comes, and we start all over again.

It's now our sixth day of climbing up and over rocks and fallen trees, dealing with insects and overall exhaustion, hiking this seemingly endless trail. Well, it's not exactly a trail, more of a path that is continually being created by Bushney, the name I gave to my new friend, as we advance through the jungle landscape.

We finally reach the summit of this unforgiving mountain range where we set up camp for the final evening before dropping off the other side tomorrow morning.

During the night, my companion fastened our ropes and harnesses for the slow descent into the forest area down the backside of the mountain. I don't think he ever sleeps, but, honestly, I haven't slept much either. Who could sleep on an adventure like this with so much to be excited for anyway?

Waking up early, I grab coffee and gently pace back and forth for some time prior to my planned departure. While waiting for the sun to rise, I simply review the course of action and make sure I have not left out any key—or even any minute—detail. Once it is time to go, Bushney properly secures the ropes to a very large stoic tree above and harnesses me in tightly.

As instructed, I begin to slowly walk backward down the side of the mountain. I had repelled various landscapes over the years, so most of this seems normal and quite comfortable. As the ropes lengthen and Bushney becomes smaller and smaller, the treetops grow in stature. It looks as if I would be landing on top of them because all that I can see below my feet is heavy branches and greenery.

As I prepare to find an acceptable landing point, I brace myself for impact, closer and closer. I'm there now, wondering if I'll have enough support to hold my body weight or if I'm going to be at the mercy of my rope skills, practicing balancing like a native tree climber until I eventually find a branched stairway down to the ground below.

Then, at the very last second, as my toes reach to gain footing, a small opening appears in the trees that could not be seen until this precise moment. Taking a deep breath and just trusting the process, I begin going through a sort of tree tunnel in the jungle, falling and falling, holding my breath and anxious until my feet are on firm ground.

As I survey the area, it's somewhat eerie, but extremely exciting at the same time. I must admit that I'm a little afraid and overwhelmed with the absolute presence of the moment. I'm just beside myself, accommodating the need to soak in the present. The culmination of so much dreaming and hoping all at the same time. Many years of anticipating this day, even on the days when some doubt crept in, and some doubt always creeps in.

Is it really there? Am I going to find what I've dreamed of for so long, or will it be another missed opportunity gone awry?

But not this time. It just feels different. It feels special. It feels right.

I've checked all of the numbers, notes, and charts time and again. I've studied the maps until they became imprinted on my brain. The measurements all match perfectly.

This is it . . .

No doubt, this is the day that I discover it! I'll get to see it. I'll get to touch it and know that it is real.

Just for reassurance, once I reach the jungle floor, I look up toward the tree tunnel I just slid down to let Bushney know that I am safely on the ground, but he is nowhere to be seen. In an effort to get my bearings, I take a quick moment to glance at my notes one last time, get down on my hands and knees, spread out the map, and take out my journal and compass. I intently follow the line already drawn out on the map from one direct point to another across the heavily treed jungle. I look up through the trees to gain as much light as possible, barely seeing the glow of the sun now rising. A sudden calm comes over me. I'm not quite sure why, but I confidently feel it.

I had been looking at all of this detailed stuff, going over the centuries-old historical records for years, looking for this long-sought-after, yet elusive, sight. But it was not needed anymore.

I stood up and just dropped it all on the ground. It wasn't necessary for me. I didn't need all of those maps and tools anymore. I'm supposed to be here. It's calling me. This is my truest destiny.

I close my eyes, lean my head back, and point it straight at the sky for a brief moment. Ready to move with my eyes still closed, I begin to walk forward and feel my way. One step, then two, then three, then another. I'm not afraid. I'm not worried I will fall into a hole in the earth, or run into a tree, or be struck by an earth crawler, like the one that made its way into my campsite and sleeping pack when traveling in Australia a few years ago. (The itchy red marks it left on my leg for several days following the attack are still vividly imprinted on my memory. I will definitely avoid repeating that experience again!) I keep walking for what feels like one hundred meters or so. Then, all of the sudden, I stop. This is it. This is the place. I'm overcome with a feeling never experienced before in my life. The best attempt at a description would be spiritual, or other-worldly. But one thing for sure, it is powerfully present and expressing itself within me.

I close my eyes, take several deep breaths, in through my nose and out through my mouth. My racing heart and the panting with excitement that plagued me thirty minutes ago are gone.

Slowly, with my eyes still closed, I lift my right hand and push aside a plant leaf the size of an elephant ear. Then I lift my left hand to push away another in the opposite direction.

As the jungle parts, I can feel a cool breeze on my face and hear water. Continuing to walk calmly and slowly, it is time to open my eyes.

Forget the calmness that I had a few minutes ago, that peaceful feeling that was so present. Now I'm in pure adrenaline mode—you know, fight or flight, heart racing full speed, breathing heavily, and even shaking a little.

Without question, this is the most anxious moment in my life. I'm now in total thrill mode and I work up the nerve to find out if all of this searching will bear fruit.

Was the pursuit of this dream really worth it, or was it another dead end, all these years of dedication a lost cause?

Treacherous and tormenting thoughts that I developed processes to deal with years ago . . . I close my eyes, take one last deep breath, and they're gone.

This is it.

I begin to open my eyes very, very slowly . . .

The light begins to crest through my barely opened eyelids. It spreads and grows, larger and larger . . . and then, my alarm awakens me.

It's 5:00 a.m.

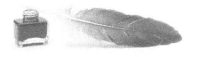

Chapter 1

BEFORE AND AGAIN

ENGLAND

While preparing for some recent travels, I made a discovery that would significantly alter my research—and overall mission—for my life's work, work I began years ago. And this discovery didn't just alter my research activity. It changed the way I understand the work, exploration, and discoveries to date, as well as, well, when it comes down to it, pretty much everything that I had learned up until that point.

To put it more bluntly—and incur some element of humility—prior to this find, I've always thought everything was on track, that the path laid out in front of me was fairly precise and accurate, that I had a fairly good handle on my pursuits as I developed sources of information, each new path moving me toward obtaining a synopsis that would prove all of the written theories. However, as it turned out, I was always a degree off here and there. Over time, those small miscalculations continued to increase until I found that my intended destination was really relatively far off course.

I have always been obsessed with understanding this thing we call life. You know, 'why am I here' and 'what is my purpose' and all that sort of stuff. That obsession and the curiosity that came with it led me to investigate many different aspects of the human experience, which led me to explore a number of possibilities, one of which was the concept of time and how time affects every experience in life.

But many things that I considered important to achieve from my labors remained elusive. I continued doing what I had always done, researching and exploring through the world of academia, as well as traveling the planet to uncover history's greatest treasures, but those efforts, although admirable and accomplished, didn't seem to make any real impact on my true goals.

I think I was starting to listen to what the world says, accepting that this was just the way things are as the years accumulated. Year by year, you get older and age, and you look, feel, and act according to those ideals, the stereotypes of existence, accepted by society. But I also really struggled with this concept. In my mind, like a lot of people, I still believed I was capable of anything. Why couldn't I live, learn, get wiser and more experienced in life, *and* still be able to do all of those awesome things that I had dreamed of doing? So, one of my major studies ended up being about understanding time. What is time? How is it calculated? Where did it begin? How do we measure it and why? What does it mean? How does it work? Could I affect it? Could I control it? Could I reverse it?

Looking back, I've always been befuddled by how humans measure time periods anyway. Seconds, minutes, hours, days, years, decades, centuries, millennia, billions of years, as the geologists proclaim, and so it goes, on and on.

Of course, there are organizational demands on our lives; arrive here at this time and deliver the item by this date, etc. However, the struggle for me was grasping how to really measure our physiology in terms of time, the body and mind, and even the soul, for that matter, as if we were a bunch of robots, literally clicking off the seconds without any control, just accepting the passing of time. Believing that's the way it is, that's the way it's always been, and that's the way it will always be. I mean, until now, my research studies concluded that time was a constant and that it impacted everyone the same way.

For instance, if you said someone is thirty years old, that conjures up a certain image in the mind, and if you say she is fifty-two years old, that's another image, and if that guy has been walking around for at least sixty-five years, yet another image is immediately registered in your brain based on what you've known and seen traditionally. But why is this? Where do those images come from? People don't look the same. They are different sizes, heights, shapes, and so on, so why would people look the same after a certain amount of clinically established time?

And that would bring me back to the universally accepted definition of time: How do you measure time anyway?

Here's what I had come to believe: At the time our mother delivers us, we start the time clock of life. Every sixty seconds, we age one minute exactly, every sixty minutes we age an hour exactly, every twenty-four hours, we age one day exactly, every three hundred and sixty-five days, we age one year exactly, and so it goes, year, after year, after year, after year.

Everyone is exactly the same. We each get the same amount of time in a minute, an hour, a day, a year, etc., and that is an accurate measure of one's life clock.

It's the same for everyone.

But is it?

Yes, numerically, it's the same, but . . . in no way do all people receive the effects of time in the same manner. Everyone does not evolve, age, or experience time the same way. In fact, no one evolves, ages, or is affected by time exactly like any other person.

If you think about it, that's kind of a remarkable statement, because there are so many factors that affect the way we experience time. Yet, we look at people all the time and wonder how old they are, or think that they look really good for their age, or think they look like time has treated them well—or perhaps not so well. Accordingly, if external effects are different, wouldn't, theoretically, internal effects be different as well?

So that got me thinking . . . what if you really could not tell what someone's life clock registry was, relative to wear and tear, etc? I mean it. What if a person could really defy the clock? What if the entire concept decided on by society at large, of numerical and chronological scoring and other stereotypical descriptions, was substituted with your physiological or real-time clock? The actual wear and tear on our person?

Then I started wondering how directly linked this alternative concept of time may be to our entire being—our organs, brain, skin, heart, liver, eyes, ears, muscles, tendons, ligaments, spirit, soul, experiences . . . every aspect of our existence.

The studies all show that there are so many factors that affect the way a person ages, their level of energy, and the health of their mind and body. The effects of the wear and tear on their human engine, so to speak.

So then my question became: What are the effects of time on a human organism and at what pace does it respond to the seconds ticking away? Is it a zero-sum game, where I am issued a life clock that is preset with a beginning and end date and just ticks away? Or a lifeline that begins in one region and works its way to another area destination that is the end of the line? Some might believe, as they look back on their lives, that these are somewhat accurate descriptions, but I'm not so sure that's true.

Of course, there are all the main factors that can affect the human organism differently, things like nutrition, activity, refreshment, sun exposure, genetics, alcohol and tobacco consumption, stress, sleep, mentality, balance, spirituality, along with so many more. Most of this information has been pretty readily available for some time.

So, my continually developing hypothesis became: What if we had the ability to change *how much* impact each of those factors had on our engine? Would it be possible to redirect the clock, perhaps even change its sphere of operation, say to age six months each year, or nine months every time the happy birthday clock struck midnight?

I think it's obvious that we can age fifteen or eighteen months each year based on many who have shown just that by how roughly they treated their engine. It's amusing sometimes how it's so easy to believe that contrarian thought, that we can age more than the measured amount of time, but it tends to be much more challenging for us to believe the opposite. How hard are we on the machines that we walk around in every day? What if it were super simple to change that process and live a totally full and complete life, pursuing every ambition, achieving all of our desires, not passing up on any dreams (in fact, enhancing them), yet be able to travel in the ultimate time machine?

The hypothesis continues that if the clock ticks off one second on our mechanized wall clock but ticks off two on our physiological body clock then it's also possible that as the clock ticks off two seconds on our mechanized wall clock, it could only tick off one second on our physiological body clock. What if it took two minutes on that same clock to represent one minute on our body and mind gauge, or two days were declared on the calendar to mark off one day on the revised life clock? What if we could literally purchase time, like a science fiction theatrical, depicting the ability to transport from one historical place in time to another through some special apparatus with lots of electricity bolts and lights and sound effects?

I know, I know, it sounds a lot like time travel in a fancy spaceship created by some unfashionable genius think tanker wearing goggles and wildly in need of a haircut, putting odd parts together in the secrecy of his garage lair. Science fiction and stories of time travel are fun entertainment, of course, but we are talking about something real, something tangible, here. A real opportunity in the life of every human being to make a choice, to defy the odds, to rewrite the rules regarding time, aging, health, illness and chronic disease, to have both time and resources to explore and experience as they choose, without traditional obstacles. The goal is not to cheat death, as you might think, but, to the contrary, to fulfill life.

Well, at least that was the theory I was contemplating when I was getting ready to go on this trip.

A little brain-strained with all the intense theorizing and in need of a break, I went back to preparing for the trip. Since I knew that I would be gone for an extended period, I was organizing all my materials and reviewing the research texts that would likely be important for my planned scholarly encounters, along with numerous published papers and diaries full of my accumulated studies through the years.

Additionally, it was necessary to reflect on some areas that I might have overlooked in the past. It's easy, really, when I get on a roll and believe the path is the correct one, to just kind of hammer down and get tunnel vision. Reminiscent of a racing horse with blinders and only one thing on their mind, continuously running toward the finish line. Nothing was going to stop this blistering thoroughbred from reaching his goal.

As a familiar tactic, tunnel vision had served me well, as I tend to finish what I start, but, in this case, there was a proverbial fork in the road and decisions to be made.

That's when I found it.

I was rifling through a number of reads in the front library of my private research sanctuary, as I call it, which had been in my family for many years lending itself to many tales of its own. The sanctuary juts out of the top side of the slopes and provides a morning view of the crisscrossing valleys far below as the sun slowly lifts from under the earth, each morning shining through the fifteen-meter windows, engulfed on the other five sides of the unusually shaped structure by more than one-hundred-meter-tall pine trees, which has always made for enjoyable and effective reading and research endeavors paired with the aroma of one of my favorite ground coffee beans. Depending on the time of year, in terms of my favorite places, it only ranks behind the extended deck from this same gallery room that lifts out over the top of the forest below. Out on the deck, you are consumed with cool, crisp air, surrounded with beauty and the sounds of nature, making it likely to find peaceful reflections each time.

Next, I spent time making sure that nothing important was missed deep in the back of the library. As I was digging behind several other books trying to find one particular text, I saw what looked like a crack in the wall. As I tried to maneuver my head and shoulders into the small area between the shelves, dust fell in my eyes as I held my breath, barely able to reach with my left index finger and peel back the crack.

After working at it for several painstaking minutes, dust filling the air in this small space and covering both me and the shelf below, the wall material broke into pieces and crumbled everywhere. I reached down to the shelf below for a towel to wipe away the debris and got a better look. There appeared to be a small hatch or door-like mechanism behind the wall of the shelf. It was dark in the confines of the crawl space, but as the dust cleared, I saw there was more, a tiny latch.

Curiosity growing, I pried open the latch of the hidden door, which was stuck, likely from years of normal house settlement or the swelling of the wood inside the bookcase. When I pulled harder, it opened with a high-pitched shrill. It was totally dark inside, but I reached into the small, wooden, square space, anxious to investigate the contents. I felt some type of bag or sack. Carefully dragging the bag out of the space, I wriggled my way back out of the cramped space between the shelves and gingerly crawled back down to the floor. Setting my new find on the center of my long, marble table, I stepped back, wiping my brow, and slipped on my glasses to take a closer look. The bag was old and white, or it used to be white, and it was about the length of my forearm, more yellowed now than white after its long residence inside a small dark tomb, the rough ribbed cloth sack tied at the opening like a sack of potatoes.

As I worked to loosen the tightly secured leather string laced up around the twisted opening, the brittle strap began to unravel, breaking into pieces. I pulled the remaining strands away from the bag, anticipation growing while I untwisted the bag. The somewhat stiff cloth created an opening, allowing me a view of its hidden contents.

Inside, there was a book.

A book I'd certainly never seen before.

It was extremely old by all appearances and in poor condition. I didn't remember possessing anything like it in my collection. I hadn't purchased it.

Where did it come from and how long had it been there deteriorating and gathering dust? Why now? What made me look there, and why did it present itself to me on this day?

It was as if it were calling out to me for help. Not for its own sake, mind you, but perhaps for mine . . .

Maybe someone or something realized that I was stumped, in need of a course correction, and in search of an answer—any answer. That someone or something pushed me, encouraged me to pursue a different direction.

You know how sometimes you feel as if something is amiss, that you're off just a little here and there? That had to be it. Whatever the reason, this slumbering storyteller decided to present itself after staying hidden for so many years. It was highly peculiar and may have been more ancient than anything I had in my possession or had even cataloged before.

What is its message, and what secrets does it hold? Who are they important to?

Well, I certainly didn't know, but I was determined to find out as I traveled across the world to visit with some of the most renowned experts in their respective fields of unique antiquities and gain some knowledge about the past year's discoveries, which had been the primary agenda; however, now I would be hoping to find some answers about this mysterious book.

What secrets it might hold and how those secrets would affect the days to follow was definitely still a mystery, but one thing was for sure: My antennas were up.

The real question was . . . what was I to do next?

To begin with, the book was in such delicate condition that I was afraid to touch it, much less open it, over concern that it might just fall apart right where it lay.

The next smart move was to call a dear friend I had known for many years. Our intellectual trust, connection, and relationship went back many years, and I believed there was no one more worthy for me to entrust this find, at this point a protected secret. She had dealt in rare artifacts for a lifetime and I felt comfortable garnering her advice and direction. At first, I involved her to make sure the book was preserved and could survive long enough to be examined, but, admittedly, I also had a grander hope that she might be able to explain what it was or maybe even take a guess at its origins. As hoped, she was gracious in accepting my invitation and would join me soon.

At an initial glance, it appeared to be written in an unfamiliar language with symbols that were unrecognizable, at least based on my knowledge. The symbols looked like some sort of hieroglyphics, an alphabet that included both logographic and syllabic elements. To say that a heightened sense of curiosity was developing would be an understatement. Sufficiently fascinated would be a better description of what I was starting to feel about this eccentric book.

For the time being, the most pressing issue was protecting this very tender item, so we first worked toward that end. My dear friend, consummate in class and elegance, a tall, slender brunette, pulled out some special tools wrapped in a leather folder tied with a cloth strap, explaining to me the delicate use of each one. It was enjoyable to watch her gently and succinctly maneuvering around her new patient with the precision of a highly practiced surgeon. She is not difficult to respect and admire with the reputation she carries as one of the world's greatest at her craft, and she was on full display. She's simply amazing.

Having painstakingly cleaned the surface and the book's edges as much as possible, the next step was to secure, actually reattaching in some cases, the material to its base. In a further effort to restore the parchment to the original state, we began a concentrated, step-by-step staged and timed process of injecting and applying various solvents, solutions, and special resins, such as polyvinyl acetate, calcium carbonate, dimethylformamide, and acrylic polymers, to secure and protect the surface prior to moving on to the final steps of restoration.

This dedicated effort is similar, although on a much smaller scale, of course, to that used by the Vatican City during its lengthy process of restoring Michelangelo's priceless work of art on the Sistine Chapel ceiling. Like that engagement, restoration was not a guarantee for us. It could possibly have done further damage to the canvas; however, we believed there was a high likelihood that it would at least give us a better surface on which to view the work.

Once sufficiently satisfied that everything had been done to ensure the safety of the book, she felt comfortable beginning the examination. After a lengthy review, she confirmed that, in fact, the language and its origin were unfamiliar to her as well. Her being a highly respected curator of antiquities recognized all over the world, this didn't sit well with her, nor did it bode well for me learning what it said. On the other hand, the brilliant professional that she is, she simply took care of the business at hand and focused on instructions for how to handle the artifact. She provided me with a specially designed container set to guarantee the book's maximum protection while transporting it during my long journey ahead. She explained that the special containers would stand firm over the expected thousands of miles, high altitudes, rough terrain, changing climates, and inhospitable conditions that it was about to encounter.

She simply called it an air compression cylinder, but it just looked like a hard, plastic encasing of some sort to the novice eye with a second outer layer to protect it. Of course, I trusted her, so I followed her every instruction to the letter, hoping to ensure the safety of the new property with which I had been entrusted.

This is where it gets really interesting.

While my friend and I were figuring out how best to touch the book and open its cover, the back tear came loose, and we saw another mystery item.

At this point, still not completely sure what it was, heart beating fast, I pulled back the vellum leaf, retrieved the hidden item from beneath the torn back cover, and placed it on my very large, leather inlaid desk, which looks like an old banker's desk, almost too big for the space in which it resides. But it's absolutely wonderful for spreading out papers or materials for in-depth examination.

Carefully, we concentrated on pulling back each fold until it was completely open and spread out, securing each edge with crystal paperweights to hold the corners down. We realigned the overhead lamp for enhanced viewing and turned the light to a brighter level to get a clearer view of the fabric. Although an educated guess at what it was had already surfaced, a much deeper examination was necessary.

Many of these archeological specialties, such as difficult-to-cipher artifacts or evolutionary efforts to communicate through figures, etchings, or drawings have been a part of my lifelong study, but this was different. Something was happening as part of a professional academic pursuit to gain answers; however, there was also something else happening at the same time. . . there's a source, a strength that is guiding me, or at least that was the sense I had. I'm not saying that the moment was easier, but I do know that the percentage of correct decisions I had made of late had increased. I seemed to end up choosing the right direction more frequently and turning over the right rocks more often than had previously been the case.

As we laid it out on the desk and adjusted the lights once again, hearts racing, breathing heavy in disbelief, we continued to fold back the paper, more like a tapestry really, with small, metal tweezers designed specifically for the gentle handling of small, sensitive objects like this one.

With a commitment to maintain its present state, we moved very slowly and methodically. As we folded back the first corner, it was unclear what it was, and the second didn't help much either, as the condition of the material was so badly worn and brittle. The damage and dust from its seclusion, along with apparent bleeding of the original inks, hid a proper view and might have ultimately obstructed the likelihood of learning anything of real value.

Once the material was completely spread out and flattened over the table, further examination began. Taking detailed journal notes, I realized it was much larger than anticipated, measuring some ninety-one centimeters across the top edge and seventy-one centimeters across the sides.

The next step was to gently clear the surface of debris and brush off the dust, which was no small task due to the fragility of . . . well, whatever it was. Carefully, we took a closer look. Thankfully there is no better person than my trusted curator to count on for dealing with these types of materials, as she had decades of experience with similar situations. Having spent years in Europe leading teams of restoration specialists in the delicate art of bringing damaged works back to their truest form. Without question, there was not a better person to have directing the work.

As I had hoped—and frankly expected—we concluded it was some sort of map, or perhaps a better description might be a protocol or outline of instructions. But of what? And why did I find it hidden in this bound manual, in a cove of the library of my home, clearly not meant to be unearthed?

Or, is it possible that it was being saved or protected from something or someone until its protector came along?

Fanciful thinking perhaps, that I might be its procurer.

Even though this appears to be a remarkable find, and it certainly would require much greater investigation, the pressing focus was not the map but the book, as I thought it might hold the answers to all of the questions that were swirling in the air.

Having complete confidence in the linguistic experts who would ultimately examine the newly encased materials, my only priority after realizing neither myself nor my friend could read it was getting it to those experts' locations without doing any further harm than the years of inactivity and slumber had already done. Patience is not a virtue of mine, for sure. Accordingly, I spent the next few days trying to get a grasp on what was in my possession, which created a great deal of anxiety for me.

After losing several days of sleep over the book that would be accompanying me on my travels, it turned out that all was not in vain. As I would soon learn, the value of its contents would not disappoint. At this stage, however, that wasn't the important part. It didn't matter what the book was worth at this point; it was only the guidance it would produce that mattered. Sure, it added to the mystery that it might be a priceless artifact or literary phenomenon, but my search for answers that the work might assist in providing was destined to be deemed truly priceless to the human race.

When originally preparing for my travels, I was planning to visit with some of the most internationally recognized archaeological experts, ancient historians, and geologists in the world about the research data I had cataloged to this point. Now these unusual relics placed themselves at the front of the line for my discussions.

My first stop was London to visit my long-time friend, who I've always simply called the Professor, at the College of History of Ancient Civilizations and Philosophy in the city's most renowned university. The Professor is actually what everyone calls him, because, frankly, anything else just seems unworthy of his stature and position. Relative to our meeting, however, he is considered one of the world's foremost experts in ancient and extremely rare artifacts, specifically rare or ancient writings and manuscripts. Being a trusted confidant, and knowing of my lifelong quest, I thought he might be as excited as I was to see what had been rescued from such an unassuming hideaway at my mountain home after so many years. I had to wonder, based on my life's pursuits, if I had found this special edition—or if it had indeed found me.

The entry to the Professor's office is unusual, to say the least. The surroundings are striking in so many ways, but not altogether unexpected. The office is dark and dreary at best. It's not actually cold, but it makes you feel that way, even with a wood-burning fireplace on the far wall and a giant, tan English Bloodhound lazily sprawled on a tightly woven antique Turkish rug just in front of the fire. It matches the classic vision that comes to mind when you think of a long-time tenured professor, tucked away in the furthest recessed basement of this two-story stone office building settled in the elm trees of the campus. There are always books everywhere without any obvious organization or structure to the process. Sitting behind his desk, there was his bearded face, a few strands of hair left on his head and horned-rimmed glasses—my long-time acquaintance, the Professor.

He got up from behind his desk to shake my hand. While I was happy to see him once again, I was taken aback by his slumped posture and the fragility of his frame as he shuffled over to give me an embrace. Time hadn't necessarily been kind to the wise old man.

After a few brief minutes of catching up on our lives and travels, like the man I had always known, he didn't waste any time getting to the point.

"Let me see it," he said.

Not surprised by his sternness, I reached into my satchel and pulled out the cylinder that had been specially designed and sealed to protect its contents.

As I gently placed it on his desk and sat down directly across from him, the Professor slowly rose back up out of his chair to examine the newly opened container, its contents still inside the inner casing. Adjusting his glasses, he began to utter sounds under his breath. The room carried the lingering odor of a pipe, which he had already reached for on the far right corner of his desk from its awkward resting place in the tray and placed gently in the corner of his mouth, grabbing it with his yellowing teeth. Still more groans, before he returned to his squeaky chair.

Interlocking his fingers, the Professor looked toward the ceiling, uttered still more groans, fingers interlocked on top of his head, and took a deep breath, seemingly troubled, or perhaps bothered. It definitely wasn't clear, and to say anything at that point would have been risky, but to not interject during the uncomfortable silence didn't seem like a great option either and left me all the more awkwardly hanging on his mutterings. So, with the perceived patience of Job, I chose the prior option and remained quiet, resting my chin on my hand, one finger draped over my mouth, looking intently and waiting.

At that point, the anticipation was nearly unbearable. What is it? What was he thinking? Was I wasting his time? Was I about to be thrown from his office? Had I upset my respected colleague?

Yes, the suspense was killing me.

Finally, he began to speak, slowly, with a slight stutter, clearly lacking confidence, and said, "I've never seen anything like this before." More groans.

Having already explained how the odd discovery was made, I did not dare respond, as surely there was more to come from my wise old friend. He leaned forward and rifled through a bunch of papers, likely prepared for our visit, strewn all over the almost unidentifiable deep dark wood platform where he spent the greater part of his years. He slowly rose from his perch and shuffled over to one of his many bookshelves.

To my amazement, he literally climbed up on a rickety tripod of a stool, extending his arm as far as he could, which was about halfway straightened, and, with his fingertips, grabbed the top edge of a binder from the middle of the bookcase. Once he had it secured under his left arm, he finally shimmied back down to the floor.

The entire experience was very intense and left a golf-ball-sized lump in my throat. Uncomfortably waiting for a possible crash of the strong-willed teacher left me rocking back and forth in my chair as the need to dart over to catch him if he fell could come abruptly. Safely back on the ground, allowing me to breathe again, and returned to the comfort of his chair, he placed the text on the muddled papers atop his desk and pressed the corners of the desk with each hand as he stood up and leaned out toward the center. After flipping numerous pages, licking his fingers after each effort, he stopped, and with a funny, wrinkled grin, said, "See, there it is."

He turned the book around toward me and gently pushed it my way. I looked intently, like a grade schooler, but I wasn't sure what I was supposed to be looking at. I just stared with a respectful focus. Sensing that I might not know what he wanted me to find, he slid his left index finger to the center of the right side of the page so I could see what his last hour of efforts had uncovered.

And there it was.

One line mentioning a reference to work done over centuries by numerous scholars from several continents, intended to share the most important finds from their respective cultures and histories.

I muttered to myself, "Okay . . . that's it? What do I do with this information?"

My old friend said, "Do you see?"

Not knowing how to respond, and not wanting to appear that I didn't appreciate his time and effort, I said, "Yes, yes, I do. However, I'm still thinking, where do I go with this information? What now?"

Much to my relief, the Professor reached into his top right-hand drawer and pulled out a notepad, leaned across the table, and wrote something on the pad, tearing it away and handing it to me. He had scribbled four letters.

I H A C

Further exploration of the Professor's mini-symposium in his office allowed me to understand what the four letters stood for: The Institute for the History of Ancient Civilizations. It was a graduate research university in the Jilin Province of Changchun, China. The institute had been conducting research positions for Assyriology, Hittitology, Egyptology, Classics, and Philology for decades. Additionally, the institute published the annual *Journal of Ancient Civilizations* that contained works by

Chinese scholars in the areas of history, art, archaeology, philology, and linguistics of the ancient Near Eastern and Mediterranean regions.

So, with the direction of my English colleague, a great deal of preparatory inquiry, adjusting schedules, rescheduling and planning, and some basic faith, my next destination was the Jilin Province of China to begin the word-by-word translation and delineation of the languages from these long-lost messengers.

Leaning back in my chair following takeoff for the ten-and-a-half-hour flight to Northeast China, I did not even see the plane reach its cruising altitude, as I was pronounced snoring prior to the landing gear being raised.

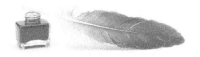

Chapter 2

THE FOUR PILLARS

ANCIENT GREECE

Arriving on the Asian continent to meet with the research scholars residing at the institute was the first step toward getting the answers I needed. Once the experts had an opportunity to examine the artifacts, the book, and the map discovered in my library, I was hopeful they would come to the same preliminary analysis that I did and take it a step further to identify the first destination of my journey.

The coordinated review with my archeologist and curator friend had led me to believe that the first entries in the book, initially analyzed in my summer research sanctuary, described an ancient script that is believed to list a series of blocks, structures, or foundations of some type. Although still a little choppy and granular, there were enough clues to determine whether it could pinpoint the first major location for uncovering a critical life pattern that may maintain some of mankind's greatest secrets.

But so many had traveled this path before me, only to come up short. Hoping that they could unveil what they believed would change mankind for all time . . . or bring us back to our original understanding of life on this earth.

You see, it's my opinion that we were meant to live forever. It's just what I've always believed. We were supposed to live, love, and pursue an eternity of existence right here on this planet we call earth. We were never meant to age, get frail, or die. We were meant to have families and relationships, pursue goals and dreams, impact our fellow man, and experience joy for all of time.

For as long as I can remember, I have had this belief, so this current path humans are on was, at best, puzzling to me. To be born, grow up healthy—hopefully—live for several decades, then begin to show signs of aging, in many cases developing horrifying diseases that might linger for many years, and then die, turn to dust, and that's it.

Perhaps I was naive, but that just didn't sound like a grand scheme to me. Hence, my developing hypothesis about time began to emerge. And that hypothesis was so grand I could rarely think of anything else. It began to consume my every waking thought. It started out simple enough as I began reading, writing, reflecting, conducting research, and inquiring from a general nature only. I consulted with respected colleagues, but I didn't share anything specific enough to reveal my master plan. Then my hypothesis just grew as it took more and more hours of each day until it was the dominant project of my research. I still had my other work, but this vision was crossing over into every project I had.

As I began to see that the current human pattern was a literal pattern for almost everyone in my life, it became quite disturbing and made me scratch my head for a while. Then, one crazy day, I wondered: Is that just the way it is? Do I have a choice? Do I have a say in the matter at all?

Thus began my lifelong research to uncover the truth about the confusing pattern of life and death, the time continuum of one's real life, if you will—Minkowski space, relativity, velocity, gravitational field, space dimensions, etc. At least, that's where it began. What a journey it has been.

Although I clearly wasn't done, I did know many things for certain, and one of them was that the life pattern I described, the typical human pattern of hoping you don't get ill before you inevitably die, is not the final answer. It is not the way it has to be or, for that matter, the way it *should be* for anyone.

My research had provided many answers that highlight my theories. I wouldn't claim to be the ultimate in knowledge or the best theorist on the subject matter; however, today many would have identified me as somewhat of an expert in this line of thinking. I didn't like to take any credit for it as almost all of the information I had accumulated was made of pieces of works created before me, by many greater minds and for many centuries. I was simply connecting the dots. But I was also very, very confident that it was, in fact, *my* role to connect the dots. To literally connect them on this mysterious map. Not that I felt chosen by anyone, but more that it was my destination, my calling. I believe that everyone has one, and this one was mine. So, in order to advance this premise, I had to be willing to follow this path wherever it led and formulate the best set of data I could ascertain and then share it with the brightest minds on this planet, allowing them to assimilate it and determine or reveal the next steps.

The scholars who have committed their entire lives to understanding and uncovering ancient civilizations, as well as many other specialists in supportive areas of study from geology, physics, archeology, history, physiology, and other immersions have become so familiar with their areas of concentration that it resembles the intimacy of family. Most of them had spent many decades of research with organizations led by teams of scholars, historians, scientists, and other highly respected academicians, completely focused and dedicated to their one specific area of expertise.

My meetings with them would test my limits, intellectually, physically, and emotionally, not to mention challenging my comprehension abilities to retain all of this information, digesting it, avoiding being distracted or overwhelmed by it, and making some really important directional decisions in the matter of just one week. If I'm being honest, the journey had already been a stretch of my brain cells as I attempted to grasp their specialties and their advanced knowledge of historical sites, their inhabitants, and the most significant events in their civilizations.

These scholars were so captivated by their one prospect of discovery and advancement of their theories that they could think of almost nothing else professionally. To say they were knowledgeable is an understatement. The work was truly personal to them, to say the least.

Some of them I had met before while working on various research projects during my travels over the years. However, some of them weren't even born when I had worked with the group before and were already considered the brightest in their fields. Regardless, I had enough connections to put these meetings together, with the Professor's help, my own personal credibility as an accomplished historian and philosopher, my research, and, frankly, the prospects of these recent discoveries. Truthfully, this factor alone was so enticing that most were going to great lengths to make sure they were included in the evaluation process. Their expectations alone added to my stress level.

However, to be perfectly honest, it was the fascination with the discovery all by itself that drew the group in. There was enough tantalizing information, including some of the writings, dating, and hieroglyphics

I shared in advance, as well as my description of the artifacts, that no true researcher interested in ancient discovery would dare pass up an opportunity to get a firsthand glance. Actually, I have to admit, to be the first to glance was a bit of a persuading element as well. It's an intellectual hierarchy status, if you will, that is enticing. Ultimately, I wanted the team to attempt to interpret what I had my hands on. Over the years, I had learned one simple truism about research: It never has a completion date. It's never really over, and one discovery leads to another, and yet another. That's the exciting—and frustrating—part of research.

With a desire to help my group of colleagues prepare, I had sent them each a letter in advance explaining the contents of my latest discovery, along with a descriptive portfolio of the artifacts themselves, including drawings highlighted with additional commentary from both my archeologist friend and the Professor.

In response, the group had divided into teams of advanced study areas, and each team had prepared a condensed catalog, if you will, for me so I could have a foundational understanding of the, in some cases, centuries or even millennia of information accumulated in the area.

To get a clear view of the sheer volume of information I had been provided in order to prepare for these meetings, you have to picture a stack of leather bound books about one meter in height. Thankfully, accompanying each study was a brief, an extensive synopsis summarizing the study of the related works. I'm really not quite sure what I would have done to prepare for the rapidly moving symposiums without those condensed outlines. The timing worked out well, as I was able to use the week prior to my visit at the IHAC to get a very, and I mean very, basic exposure to each of the areas of study. Being prepared for the next week involved several late nights. I had to get through each of the catalogs, make my own notes, and create a list of critical questions and a historical event order of each outline. Oh my, I wasn't sure one week would be enough time, but I gave it everything I had.

With one last evening to fine-tune everything for my first meeting at the Institute, I was miraculously ready. I might even have been a little overprepared, if there is such a thing. If only my old college history professor, whom I adored, could have seen me. Soon to be surrounded by a team of brilliant—not a term used lightly, I mean, truly elite, blow-your-mind—scholars in their respective fields of concentration, I was clear-minded and raring to go.

Each meeting, all completely different and specific in nature, would be informative and enlightening. They were exactly what needed to be done to draw closer to the answers I was pursuing. The wealth of information that was being coordinated on that site offered the opportunity to really break through the chasm that had stumped me for so long. I was determined to get every ounce of clarity I could, no matter the wear and tear on my mind, body, and spirit. I wanted to know that I gave it my all when I looked back many years after.

It was very early Monday morning, at 4:03 a.m., to be exact, and sleep wasn't much of an option. I was feeling overwhelmed and was anxious to meet my first team and its leader, the illustrious and renowned expert in all things archeological. He was perhaps the most recognized and famous archeologist in the world. I pulled together all of the related materials and stuffed them into my satchel. From what I had heard and understood from the host's remedial introduction, this particular expert, whose reputation proceeded him, was known for a directness that is . . . less than welcoming, so I didn't want to bring any of that attention toward me by being late or unprepared.

I needed some coffee.

I settled down at my makeshift hotel office to organize my notes once again. I thought I was ready to go, but I wanted to get one last review.

At that point, listening intently, taking notes, and asking relevant inquiries seemed the way to go. The night before, I had compiled a list of questions that would hopefully get me the information and guidance I needed to successfully launch the next leg of this journey.

When we go through certain types of challenges in life, they can seem insurmountable. However, isn't it comforting to know that when we get through them and look back, as difficult as they may have seemed at the time, we are always stronger? We come to realize that we really can make it to the other side if only we just keep moving forward.

I was a little nervous about that first meeting, of course. That's to be expected. But for some reason, I was also doubting my own abilities and feeling rather underqualified to be in my position. However, I just kept telling myself that if I kept taking small steps forward with faith, I would eventually find a clearer path, and this would be no different.

When I walked into the first conference meeting, I didn't know what to expect. It was a normal conference setting like most offices have, with a long table and about twenty chairs surrounding it. I'm not sure what I was expecting—maybe a table full of genius types—but to my surprise, the room was empty other than one person, a gentleman sitting in the last chair along the side of the long conference table, slumped over his notebooks. He was maybe sixty years old by appearance with a scraggly beard. He was dark-skinned, perhaps Middle Eastern of origin, but I couldn't be sure.

I walked over to him, introduced myself, and told him what an honor it was to meet him and how much I appreciated him taking the time to meet with me.

It wasn't completely clear if he had actually prepared for the meeting, as it just seemed second nature to him to disclose with total confidence what he believed my next step needed to be.

Of course, I needed to understand more about what brought him to that conclusion. He had been provided an analysis of my global plan and my overall intent of discovery. It was thorough, but my mission was at somewhat of an impasse and obviously needed direction in order to continue.

It did not take long to find out that the famed archeologist was, as described, a man of few words, and it was for certain that he had done his homework and was thoroughly prepared. Without even introducing himself and with a prideful crassness, he abruptly exclaimed, "Greece! You must go to visit the Ancients. There you will uncover what you are looking to find."

He continued to indoctrinate me on his favorite subject: Greece is officially the Hellenic Republic, known as Hellas in Southeast Europe, with a population of more than ten million people and Athens being the largest, and capital city, with Thessaloniki following as the next largest. Sitting on the tip of the Balkan Peninsula, Greece is the crossroads of Europe, Asia, and Africa. Eighty percent of Greece is mountainous, with Mount Olympus being the highest peak at over 2,900 meters above sea level. Today, all of Greece is a popular travel destination; however, Greece is also considered the cradle of Western civilization, being the birthplace of democracy, Western philosophy, Western literature, historiography, political science, major scientific and mathematical principles, Western drama, and, of course, the Olympic games.

The archeologist went on and on, not just describing the country as it currently was, but addressing more specifically the Dark Ages of the Greeks from the twelfth to the ninth century BC through circa AD 600, which was the end of antiquity. The influence of the classical Greek culture had a significant impact on ancient Rome and the Mediterranean Basin and throughout Europe, becoming the seed of Western culture. It is for this reason that Classical Greece is considered the cradle of Western civilization, emphasizing the importance of the pursuit of knowledge.

"So," he concluded, "You must go there now to get your answers."

Of course, I would have liked to do that very much, but given that I'm an overly detailed researcher and that it was only the first day of many similar meetings, and that meeting was just addressing the first entry in the book (the one with which the brilliant archeologist was familiar), I couldn't leave immediately. There were several more writings to learn about before I could put the puzzle pieces of the map together with any confidence.

After eight days of more of the same kinds of meetings, I was exhausted and felt like I could probably sleep for a week, but there was no time for that.

The wonderful news was that these talented scholars had developed into a team and worked so willingly together, even though they came from different backgrounds, possessing different views on almost everything with an affinity toward the works they had spent much of their lives understanding. Even though they were so committed to their specific concentrations and had obvious biases, all of the group members coordinated their efforts toward finding the answers set out in my developing theories. As the pieces of these complex and highly sophisticated historical explorative journeys crossed paths, it became clear that four of the studies were going to be an integral part of my specific search and next steps.

With the initial conferences complete, extremely detailed data accumulated, and what I believed wholeheartedly to be a firm action plan in place for how to move forward, the outline for the first of several destinations was constructed. This was the beginning of a very long and trying expedition for sure, but it would be well worth it.

I had previously traveled to Greece for a more relaxing experience, but this time it would be different. This time was going to be a haul, and, at this point, I was in a highly focused and driven mode, almost numb, barely-feeling-my-face type of space. It may have been complete euphoria, exhaustion, or mental deprivation, but interestingly, I had achieved some sort of belief that I was prepared to handle whatever might come.

There came a point when I was pressed so far I thought: Bring it on. What else can you do to me? I've been through so much in my life. I can deal with this too.

I had felt that way a couple of times before, so I was quite familiar with what it feels like. It's somewhere between 'I don't care anymore' and 'I'm too tired to feel anything anyway, so go ahead and take another whack at me.'

Of course, I really did care, but it's an interesting state to be in when you say to yourself: I'm not listening to you anymore. I'm not listening to the doubters. I'm on a mission, and everyone else will just have to live with it, and so will I—no matter the cost.

In many ways, that mental space is actually quite liberating for the psyche. I wanted to stay there for a while and just breathe it in. It's a flow, a rhythm that keeps me on course. I certainly am not in that space continually, but when I am, it can be extremely rewarding. Yes, I like it, the freedom of expression and peacefulness. A complete confidence really.

After I arrived in Athens, looking forward to pursuing the dossier provided me by the famed archeologist, I dove into his prepared information. The narrative was that the Ancient Greek civilization would apparently lead to four stones that explained knowledge, science and religion, mathematics, and philosophy and would hopefully open the door to a different set of structures that formed the foundational basis of all my years of research.

Traveling back in time to this place classically considered to be the cradle of Western civilization engaged a certain level of imagination as I grasped for a vision of my exploration now underway. Illuminated by my surroundings, my excitement continued to grow with the contemplation of actually making a real, identifiable step toward my destiny. I saw the stones I was seeking as pillars, much like those at the Parthenon, a temple dedicated to Athena located on the Acropolis in Athens, which obviously is one of the most recognized and representative symbols of the culture and sophistication of the ancient Greeks.

Even the Mediterranean Sea in and of itself was magical and mystical. History has lingered on its shores for centuries, along with dramatic Greek lore, creating great works of art, literature, culture, discoveries, social presence, and so much more. It can be overwhelming if you let it, but I had learned better. I knew I must focus on the task at hand to uncover the instructions locked away by time for a path toward a better understanding of human design.

The first direction provided by the archeologist was to find the ancient key, long thought to be in the annals of Pytho, containing the inner sanctum of Pythia's reliquary. Pythia was believed to be the guide of ancient Greeks and to live at the center of the world in Delphi, as it was to be later known. Delphi is located along a slope range of mount Parnassus and is held to be the sanctuary of Apollo, the Greek god of knowledge, light, and harmony. This semicircular spur is known as Phaedriades and overlooks the Pleistos Valley.

My search began at the base of the Omphalos, which is translated to mean navel, an ancient stone baetylus believed to be sacred and blessed with life. According to Greek lore, Zeus sent two eagles from opposite ends of the world at the same time, flying at an identical pace in expectation that they would cross each other's path at the exact center of the world. When they met above its center at Pythia, Zeus granted this spiritual site a stone monument, declaring it the most significant place in the world.

The climb that was in front of me was significant and I expected it to take several weeks, as the ancient valley of Phocis was massive, covering more than 965 kilometers with the elevation to reach the plateau of Mount Parnassus in excess of 2,400 meters. That was all well and good, as they say. The journey is the best part anyway, and I was prepared to tackle this breathtaking monument.

The view as my guide and I approached the base was magnificent. The ridge of Parnassus covered the clouds and it appeared as if I could reach up and grab them once the ascent had been achieved.

After about six days of climbing, I was blistered and in need of a bath, but I had also become somewhat accustomed to that way of life. I'm always amazed by what the human mind, body, and spirit are capable of enduring. I've come to believe that almost anything can be obtained with diligence toward a truly desired end.

The ascension to the peak of Mount Parnassus was strategic, of course, not just an attempt to crest another landscape. You see, this was where an ancient Greek historian at the institute, in support of the archeologist's outline, believed that Cronus, the ruler of the mythological Golden Age, was told by Pythia to hide the first ancient key, as Parnassus was derived to mean, 'the mountain that is the house of the god.'

Early the seventh morning, I crested the mountain top. The plan was to reach and stand firmly on the summit before the sun rises to experience the light as it first shines on the mountain, exactly as it had done for thousands of years.

As I traversed the area outlined by the delicately detailed map and accompanying instructions, I came to the upper eastern corner of the plateau where the configuration of stone images was drawn on the map. As I looked between the drawing and the physical landscape, it was uncanny how accurate the map read. I walked up to the area as it instructed, looking for a mountain-goat-shaped rock image with golden flamed wings and horns. It took a little imagination, but I was able to get there. As I curved around to the backside of the stone structure, to my amazement, there was a ledge leading down the slope of the mountain, so I descended very carefully. It was a circular staircase, a stone path about fifty meters long onto the internal slope of the mountainside.

As I descended, I came to a natural landing, and there it was as described: the four pillars approximately six meters in height, heavily worn and damaged from the wear of time as one might expect. It was somewhat of an eerie sight, almost ghostly, as a very cool breeze and the accompanying whistle overwhelmed the very place where they were erected. I didn't feel alone. It's as if someone else was there, watching over the space and its secrets. I wanted to respect the sight and the moment, but I was also anxious to gain the knowledge I needed and continue on my journey. They had to possess the key. After hours of searching, I discovered that, whatever key was there (which I now believe to be a manuscript or engraving of some sort) had been removed; however, having been there for many hundreds of years, as presumed, it left an impression of the drawings or etchings in the structure itself. The archeologist believed, and after seeing the display, so did I, that it was the first ancient key. It was always described at the institute as the missing piece to uncover the lost words of Apollo; yet, in those drawings was the message of Apollo to his kingdom.

The carvings and artifacts would obviously need much further examination by the experts at the institute, as well as the new councils being formed in Switzerland and America. They conveyed the message of Apollo's competitions and the story of him being speared by the horn of a boar while hunting. He had slain a giant Python and later the spot would become the home of the Pythian Games. Greeks from all over the land would come to compete for the Stephanos, a laurel crown cut out of a tree by a boy who performed the ceremonial slaying of the python by Apollo, and ultimately be named the victor of the games.

The Greek competitors were committed to their craft. They were focused on the four pillars of ultimate athleticism: activity, nutrition, rejuvenation, and balance. They had a dedication to proper nutrition in order to fuel their bodies for performance and the ultimate training, strength, and conditioning regimen to ensure peak performance. In an effort to stay on track for their competitions, they would refresh their bodies and minds so they could arrive at their premium height of performance when needed. The key was complete when the athletes had also achieved a platform of spiritual illumination, transforming their mind, body, and soul to a higher level of esteem. This find was exhilarating but required greater clarity.

Following my trip to the ancient civilization of Greece, loaded with a host of information, I found myself called to visit a long-time friend and confidant who had spent his entire life attempting to scientifically draw the lines between the special gifts we are born with and the modern-day medical treatments and processes we have come to rely on. It was his mission. Holding several degrees with a leading concentration for most of his research in biochemistry, he had published many works on related subjects. After decades of becoming highly accomplished in this line of thinking, he knew that to make an impact and continue to be accepted in the greater annals of higher thinking, he needed to coordinate with a renowned medical expert, which is exactly what he did, teaming up with a universally recognized medical professional who concentrated in diseases of the heart and brain. As fate would have it, these two great minds in the science and medical worlds would be speaking together during my scheduled return to London.

We had already set a meeting to discuss my findings from the Ancient Greece site; however, I was also going to have the pleasure of attending their latest colloquium, and I couldn't be more excited to listen to their findings, as well as see the approach to the analysis of the recently combined data.

Entering the old building on the university campus, I knew I was in for a treat. The place was packed with young, bright, energetic minds yearning to hear from these giants of scholarly accomplishment in their respective fields. There was not a seat to be had, so I just slipped in through the back doors and found a spot to lean against the wall and await what was likely to be an enlightening evening.

As my friend walked on stage to applause and plenty of yelps, it brought back many memories from some years ago. A lot of wonderful themes were discussed in his talk, but I was mostly interested in the very specific areas of application that applied directly to my continued research and, more specifically, to my most recent trip and latest discoveries. The giant whiteboard, with handwritten scribbling that only academics can pull off, was filled with medical and scientific terminology. If you were not highly sophisticated in the field and present the entire evening, you would likely not know what any of the instructions meant.

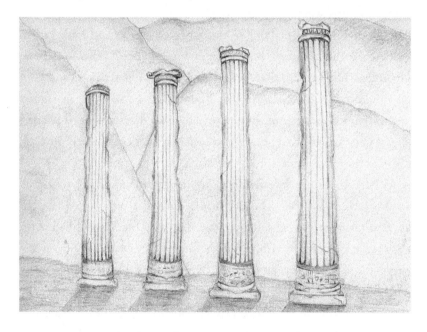

They had listed all kinds of scientific jargon and not-easy-to-grasp words like mitochondria being the powerhouse of the cells, epigenome recording of the chemical changes to the DNA and histone, sirtuin genes, influencing cellular processes like aging, etc., DNA (one I recognized), nicotinamide for metabolic processing of nutrients, adenosine triphosphate that provides energy toward driving living cells, PGC1 and FOXO 1 and 4 regulating genes involved in energy metabolism, and nicotinamide riboside claiming to be some new form of vitamin B, hypothalamus, NF-kB effecting cytokine and cell survival, and on and on it went.

I just didn't see the need to be that complicated. I'm more of the mind: Just give me the facts and tell me what it does for me. I truly think that they simply get so excited expressing their research and excellence in academics that sometimes they get lost in the moment sharing what they care about deeply. However, no one could deny the passion or the dedication that went into their work.

Oh, and they also had BDNF, or Brain Derived Neurotrophic Factor, written on the board, which is a protein generated from additional blood flow to the brain that feeds the growth of blood vessels and even new brain cells. That was kind of illuminating, actually. Their studies are fascinating and encouraging, especially with them now coordinating efforts to bridge the gap between science and medicine, which provides the next on-ramp to advance my research.

I have to admit, I really do enjoy being in the world of tenured academicians. It's full of fascination and discerning minds with an endless amount of energy. And the audience was filled with those minds, hanging around with lots of questions following the completion of the formal lecture (those inquiry sessions are usually where the good stuff happens anyway with answers that aren't usually addressed during the prepared presentations). So, in short, this is just how academic intellectuals prefer to communicate, which was fine, and I respect their intellectual exuberance of course, but I wanted to know the bottom line, as well as some very specific answers that I desperately needed.

Having known the speakers and followed their careers for years, I decided to stick around to see if they might be available to grab a cup of coffee and visit for a few minutes. That was my pitch, at least. It never hurts to ask, I always say. Accordingly, we did get to have that chat, catching up on each other's career, life, and travels, eventually getting around to the topic at hand, which was my desire to break down the topics of the evening's deliberation into a very simple layman's explanation.

I continued to inquire, asking probing questions and listening intently, which I haven't ever been very good at but have learned the benefits of over the years, we finally got around to some clearer responses, which more succinctly reflected the four pillars that led to optimal human organism functioning, as I eventually termed them. The first pillar was about the history of movement on the assets of the body and mind and how it impacts the resulting strengths and weaknesses in a great number of areas. The second was a look into the effects of what the body consumes on a consistent basis, from air to nutrients, then another relating to rejuvenation, a sense of constant natural rebuilding or reformation, and the final pillar being the ability to coordinate and balance all of these elements effectively throughout one's life with the theoretical intent to operate the organism as optimally and efficiently as it was originally designed and constructed.

I began to realize that these ancient civilizations, as we call them, may actually have been very similar to our lives today, from their diets and food sources to their daily activities lived by design. They may have understood—and were complete and totally satisfied with—what life had given them while they lived. It was exactly what they needed and nothing more. It's interesting how much the human body, brain, and spirit act similarly. When they receive the correct amount of nutrients, activity, refreshment, and balance, they respond accordingly, generating greater efficiency, energy, strength, and rejuvenation, while the mind thinks more quickly and clearly.

These idealized, yet resourceful conversations led me to recall a quote from one of the greatest minds in history: Hippocrates.

"If we could give every individual the right amount of nourishment and exercise, not too little and not too much, we would have found the safest way to health."

Certainly, this had to be a formula to obtain more fulfillment and joy from your life. And if the formula exists, what would be of greater value to possess? And what lengths would I go to obtain it?

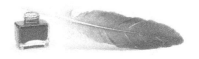

Chapter 3

DATING ADVICE

THE MAYA CIVILIZATION

Climbing to the top of the mountain was no small feat. It was over 4,300 meters to the summit of the volcano, but first I spent several days traversing the river systems, which is some 250 kilometers in length. The rivers move at a constant pace, but, for the most part, are not dangerous. The entire experience was more of a test of will than concern of actual danger, although there were some stressful moments early on as I tossed and turned up toward the Yucatan peninsula.

Being in an original cradle of civilization requires little imagination. I instantly believed that it was no normal location.

By definition, as one might expect, a cradle of civilization is a place where the birth of a civilization began, much like Greece is considered the cradle of Western civilization. And civilizations are defined as having various attributes that identify them, including agriculture, buildings, writing systems, animal husbandry, architecture, a system of classes, cities, and other public facilities.

It is believed that the original cradles of civilization developed independently and that there was not one single cradle, although the Fertile Crescent, which was Ancient Egypt, Mesopotamia, Ancient India, and Ancient China are considered to be the first. Most scholars agree that the civilizations of Mexico and Norte Chico, in the north central region of Peru, evolved separately from the Eurasian civilizations in what is considered Mesoamerica.

It has been long and well thought that the Maya civilization was one of these original cradles. There was something unusual in its midst . . . unlike many of the others that sprouted up around the world, it was on a continent all alone. The others were in what is now modern-day Europe, or the Middle East, or Asia. The most impressive achievement of the civilization was its monumental architecture, including large earthwork platform mounds and sunken circular plazas. Archaeological evidence suggests the use of textile technology and, possibly, the worship of common god symbols, both of which recur in pre-Columbian Andean cultures. It's assumed that a sophisticated government was required to manage this culture, but questions remain over the government's organization, particularly the influence of food resources on politics. During the decline of the civilization, canals developed to the north as the people were forced to migrate toward more promising fertile lands, where they could use their knowledge of irrigation to cultivate the region.

Why and how did these people get there, and how did they not only survive but thrive as they did? What was the formula for success that allowed them to develop such an accomplished way of life?

I had read many tales of this land; however, I'm not sure any of the tales did it justice toward describing the true and natural beauty, the serenity, and the feeling of being perfectly isolated. The isolation did not feel like a bad thing somehow; it was more a sense of being okay alone—or even lost—for once, not really concerned about anything. As if it was my last destination on earth, and I knew everything would be just fine. I had never felt that way before, never having completely just let go to utterly be in the present without great effort. I could experience everything completely. I could feel my lungs breathing, my heart beating. I could see everything. The colors were so powerful, affecting my senses so completely that it was as if I had painted them myself. My vision was clear.

As I looked around at the vastness of the topography, it was all-consuming, but I wasn't fearful. It was as if I belonged, as if the jungle accepted me.

No, more than that—it was as if it was protecting and guiding me.

It became calmer as the darkness arrived and the waters stilled as if they feel it too. If there were any great dramatics to come later, they could wait. I was at peace. I belonged here—not yesterday or tomorrow, but in that very moment in time—and I was okay.

That peace provided me the control to be 'here and now' in that moment. I wasn't sure when I last slept, but wasn't tired at all. I doubted I would sleep that night. I was so alive and in touch with that lost, rarely visited, hidden universe. No one else was here, and I expected no human contact for several days . . . but I didn't feel alone as the elements offered perfect companionship.

That night, I was fulfilled by enjoying what had been given me. The next day, I would climb.

Getting an early start, I was ready to go. I had all the proper gear of course. Being neither a novice nor an expert, I had a respect and reverence for the terrain as it unfolded in front of me. I walked for about five hours just to get to the base of the volcano, and when it was time to ascend, I had to look straight up at the great presence standing right in front of me as the behemoth structure that it had grown to be was daunting, yet satisfying, to view.

The terrain treated me fairly as I began the ascent. I could handle climbing for many hours, as physically preparing for these ventures had been a lifelong conditioning pattern of mine. I've always believed in adding just one element at a time to gain strength, only moving to the next once that element was conquered. After six hours of driving straight up the mountain without a break, I reached a plateau from which I could see the landscape below, as good a place as any to rest, hydrate, and take in some nourishment. As I turned to appreciate my accomplishment of making it halfway to the peak, I scanned the vast landscape, looking slowly from left to right, not wanting to miss anything. I was taken back from this massive visual, the sight encompassing all of my senses, much like when I initially viewed this terrain before my climb. I couldn't breathe, but I also couldn't stop breathing with anticipation of the sight and the anxiousness about what was to come. All I could do was simply lift my arms, fully extended out to the sides in awe of this view.

Who made this land, and how has it stayed so pure and seemingly untouched for all of this time?

Well, I knew part of the answer.

Since this land is part of a chain of volcanoes spread out along the Pacific Coast, stretching along the Central American Isthmus, extending from Guatemala, El Salvador, Honduras, Nicaragua, and Costa Rica, all the way down to northern Panama, it's called the Central American Volcanic Arc, often referred to as CAVA. This line of volcanoes reveals hundreds of formations that outline the varying types of volcanic experiences from centuries of activity, including the always enticing lava domes, cylinder cones, and stratovolcanoes of hardened lava, tephra, pumice and ash, and other clear reminders of the ferociousness of volcanic eruptive activity through the ages.

The volcanoes that are part of the CAVA are strewn over more than 1,500 kilometers and have been formed by an active subduction zone along the western boundary of the Caribbean Plate. One of the violent eruptions that carved the landscape was the Santa Maria volcano of 1902, which recorded an enormous explosion. Some of the other volcanoes in the CAVA region that are still active today are Arenal, Poás, and Rincón de la Vieja in Costa Rica; Cerro Negro, San Cristóbal, Concepción in Nicaragua; Chaparrastique or San Miguel, Ilamatepec or Santa Ana, Izalco in El Salvador; and Santa María or Santiaguito, Pacaya, Fuego in Guatemala. Actually, there are volcanos in Guatemala that reach higher than any others in Central America, which includes the Tajumulco and Volcán Tacaná that reach more than 4,000 meters toward the heavens.

I needed to keep moving to stay on track for my scheduled arrival at the summit, but for some reason, I had to take in that brief moment and determined that I could make up the time on the next leg of the climb.

Several more hours of climbing passed and despite all the physical training, I was at my last ounce of strength. As if I was writing my own script, allowing just enough words to tell the story that would accomplish the task at hand and no more, there appeared a brief glimpse of what looked to be the top. On cue, my adrenaline spiked as if I had just woken up fresh and rested for the day's adventures. (It's amazing how the soul's hope breeds strength in the physical body.) My pace increased, and I marched up that mountain as if it were my very own perfect line that I had memorized and ascended many times before.

Finally, after two more hours, the ridge of the summit appeared, and I broke into a full sprint. I jumped up to the ledge and crested over the final edge. Exhilarated at reaching the summit, I fell on my hands and knees—not from a feeling of exhaustion, but because I was thankful for another objective realized.

I took a few minutes to get some air. I was not simply out of breath; the air felt different. I had never taken in oxygen like that before. It was as if it was from another place, whatever that means . . . The air was so crisp and plentiful and seemed to go on forever. I felt I had never held that much air in my lungs before.

Standing upright, I faced the darkening blue sky as night approached, spanning toward eternity, filled with stars so bright and clear that I could count each one individually. I moved very slowly in a circle with my arms stretched out to my sides as far as I could reach looking upward, accompanied by foreverness in every direction, staring at the endless night.

I saw the early sky and stars above and ancient forestation below as far as the eye could see as they melted into the shadows. It was official. I would camp there under the scenic, endless greatness and dream of where tomorrow would lead.

That night under the stars I would also hope for answers. I would hope that I would be granted much greater clarity because the whole purpose for this climb was to find the secret that the institute believed held answers to the map I had discovered. Of course, I wanted nothing greater than to find that secret as it still appeared to be a mirage.

All of the sudden, a roar reached out and startled my senses. I reconnected to the present moment and recognized that it was thunder booming out of nowhere. It sounded far off in the distance at first but rapidly grew nearer to the campsite until it was precisely above me, like a silo outlining my body, descending from the center of an orchestrated symphony delineated directly down toward my eyes as I laid on my back in peaceful reverence.

Usually, you know when there is going to be a storm by recognizable indicators. The temperature cools, there is some light wind at first, clouds forming, barometric pressure rising, sounds of the sky beginning to drum; however, the storm didn't give me any warning at all. It was just the opposite. The sky started to rumble very gently, as if it was speaking directly to me. Like a virtuoso stroking a brilliant work and stringed instruments spinning a gentile chorus. Calmly, I listened as if it were a messenger from above, hoping it was telling me that I was on the verge of something magnificent, heading in the right direction, the path toward completion was in sight and I should forge ahead. That I should be calm and carry on. Not one drop of rain presented itself as the thunderous lullaby lulled me into a deep sleep, allowing the first restful night I could remember in a long time.

Just like so many answers that come in life, the answer that came to me was not obvious to the human eye and psyche. I spent the next few days searching for an answer, a clue, a physical identifier of some sort. A marking or carving left behind by the ancients directing me to the next phase of my exploration. (I knew that ultimately I would be obliged to make the next giant maneuver myself, but physically tracking history like this does involve outlining each step of exploration as concisely as possible.) It was only after exhausting every ounce of energy I had left, turning over every stone, and reaching a stage of wanting to give up that I realized the answer I sought was right in front of me the whole time.

I always believed that if I wanted something enough, I could make a decision and just go get it, and there is some truth to that declaration. However, it's not always that easy, or perhaps rarely is it that easy, since truly great things only come from overcoming great obstacles. This would be no different, as the simplest answers often are the most difficult to find. I think that may just be how humans work.

The other concentration I have, which I have found to be important and intertwined with the core of my life research, is the psychological realm. Obviously, this can be more difficult to grab hold of in some instances, but it affects—or perhaps even controls—the physical elements whether we are tuned into it or not.

For instance, I've always been intrigued by the notion of New Year's resolutions. I remember a different night . . . It was December 31, New Year's Eve, and I had so much to do that day. It was the last day of the year and, of course, I would be celebrating like most people. What else do you do in the final hours of the year? It's a final exuberant annual release of expression. Everyone is at this similar place and time together, which generates some peace. However, unlike most other holidays and celebrations, it is overtly jubilant while time is standing still for the whole world during that final countdown.

It always felt like a balancing act, thinking of the previous twelve months and the new twelve months ahead—the past and the future, what I had learned and accomplished, what I had experienced, and what possibilities and challenges were ahead. Like straddling a boundary line between two countries, right on the marker where an invisible line has been drawn to determine when you leave one and enter another. Literally being in two separate places at the same time. It seems a little silly and confusing to be in two places at one time, but there I am.

That's how the new year feels. It feels like I'm leaving behind the adventures of the past and stepping into the dreams of the future at the same time. Some nostalgic emotions arise for sure, along with the excitement of what is to come.

Isn't that an interesting dichotomy?

To begin new chapters of my life and see where they will take me, or to build on the wonderful ones already written, sounds fascinating. However, I have to admit, even though the excitement for the future is always real, I can never escape the melancholy hanging over me. The back and forth is probably normal, but both always seem to grab at me.

Have you ever been at a fork in the road like that in life? Where you're comfortable because you are among the familiar, whether the familiar has been easy or hard? It's comfortable because you know it very well, so you know there won't be many surprises. It's like a family member or a friend you've known your whole life; they may drive you nuts at times, but you still love them and can relax around them. You may need some time to yourself, but you also know that's still the best place for you because you know exactly where you are and what to expect.

The other is the unfamiliar, where you don't know what to expect. What will the future hold? Will it be difficult? Will you long to go back to the familiar?

But on that same side of the coin, the unfamiliar, is also the great unknown, the untraveled paths. A universe of the unsure, filled with excitement. What does it have in store for me? How can I know? I can lay out a game plan that has dates and expectations, a real list to follow, but you're never really sure how life will turn out or which roads will call your name. It takes a lot of guts and a little faith to step off the shore and sail into the wild blue, but I think that's the stuff that makes life super interesting too.

As all of this contemplation takes residence, once again, maybe I don't want to say goodbye to the familiar, maybe I want to keep it around for a while. Could I have just another thirty days? I'm not sure whether the next steps will be wonderful or extremely difficult. Then again, maybe I'm ready to say goodbye to this year and build on what I've achieved, or perhaps the past year has been a real pain. Each year brings a little of both I think. And so the back and forth goes.

As for the New Year's celebration, it is an annual tradition for me, with all the excitement and jubilant expressions it brings. It's a refreshing new start. The weather is cold, and it's an occasion to get dressed up, so I wear festive clothes, maybe a scarf and gloves, a coat, and even my freshly polished leather boots. Getting all spiffed up to ring in the new year is a fun experience. I have a glass of champagne perhaps and experience holiday cheer for everyone. There will be family and friends, excitement and fun. The elation of the evening is palatable. Who doesn't enjoy 'out with the old and in with the new,' kissing those you love, and feeling hope for the future all around?

There is so much optimism in the air. You can actually feel it. It's a physical presence, so tangible you can reach out and grab it. Pumped for the evening, I always wonder: Shouldn't I feel like this all the time? Why is everyone in such a good mood anyway? Is it just the chance to join in the crowd and truly let your hair down for an evening? The entire world agrees that this night should be jubilant and joyous just for a date change. Is it the belief in the future and, more importantly, in feeling the right now? Catching that magic moment in time that is truly tangible directly on this occasion and no other? Why does this night provide such clarity? The midnight chorus strikes the same way every midnight hour, so what makes this one different from any other?

It just feels right. It seems right. How do I capture this feeling in a bottle and sell it? If I could, I'm sure I could get a pretty penny.

Perhaps the feeling comes from the congratulatory experience between friends and peers on a job well done or dreams realized during the year. Maybe some memorable event happened during the year—getting married, the birth of a child, or a personal achievement. It may just be a relief to have made it through the year. We survived another one.

Regardless, New Year's Eve never fails to deliver an exuberant celebration across the globe.

And when I think of the new year, all of the memories of the past year come to mind for me—the movies that touched my life, a sporting event, national events that affected how I saw the world or myself in the world. Maybe it was a song or a relationship or an experience with my career that will make for a brighter future or help me evolve toward my ultimate life goals in the year to come.

However, just as well, there's always the chance that my celebration may be an expression of relief that I made it. You can say whatever you want, but I made it through the year. I survived one more time.

I hope it's the former, a hopeful celebration for the future and the accomplishments of the last year, but both feelings have their place and provide an understanding in which to reflect upon.

More importantly, what is it about this day that brings up the exuberant feeling of hope and nostalgia? Why do we wait until each year is almost over to experience such hope and optimism? Is it something that we learned, a habit we've just become accustomed to? What makes this date any better than another for us to decide what we're going to do?

I guess it's better to have a predetermined reset date than no reset date at all, or to just procrastinate resetting, delaying again and again.

And every year, I'm sure that I'll get asked ten times if I've made New Year's resolutions yet, and even though I've already been thinking about them for a while, I'm never sure I want to share them with anyone. I never know if they really care anyway, or if it's just polite conversation, like asking how it's going or how someone's weekend was. It's not that people don't really care—they might—but generally, those questions are just a way to initiate a conversation or be social.

That question does always give me pause though because I'm no longer even sure that setting New Year's resolutions is a good idea anyway. It's just something I've always done. I mean, who made up this rule that we were going to be ready to start something new or change our path on this predetermined day each year? Seriously, what's wrong with February 12 or May 19? Those dates seem as appropriate for a reset as any other.

Is it because we are turning over the calendar and a new year is starting? Or is it truly just a habit no one has thought to question?

Regardless of why, I always feel I must set new goals, set dates and make plans, and then share with everybody. So, I find myself asking: What will be on my list this year? If I share my goals, will everyone be watching to see if I actually come through and deliver on them?

As we draw closer to midnight each year, I anticipate singing in unison a Scottish poem from 1788, set to the tune of a traditional folk song, "Auld Lang Syne," breaking out into cheer, and bidding farewell to the old times to ring in the new.

Ten, nine, eight, seven, six, five, four, three, two, one . . .

Happy New Year!

Joy, kisses, and hugs all around the room.

So now, in the age-old tradition of New Year's and new beginnings, we participate in setting our New Year's resolutions. Everyone is in the same place—a new year and fresh start, a new beginning for every human being on this planet. Lined up waiting for the race to begin as the gun is fired and off we go racing down the track.

And the New Year's resolutions usually go something like this: I am going to lose weight. I am going to read more. I am going to work out every day. I am going to be a better spouse, a better friend, an altogether better person. I am going to go to church more often. I am going to make more money, get out of debt, improve my financial situation, be positive, help someone, serve a charity or my community, advance or go in a different direction with my career, etc, etc.

All that sounds pretty fantastic.

But what would that actually look like? I could make a goal to read more books, say two per month, or be a better person, be a better friend, spend more quality time with loved ones, or get in shape and be more fit. I could plan to have more quiet time and less stress or make more money and improve my financial position. All of those sound reasonable. Oh yeah, and I could also decide to eat healthier, give up alcohol, or not eat bad carbs, or give up late-night snacking.

As with any clinical trial, the experiment would be formal, setting out the parameters, input, controlled and uncontrolled elements of the environment, a hypothesis with theoretical outcomes, antecedent, assumptions, sample and data analysis, and conclusions adopted. The test subject would be weight loss and increased fitness. Considering that one of the most popular annual goals is to lose weight and increase fitness, that substratum became the test proof for determining the effectiveness of New Year's resolutions toward that outcome.

The research question: Does beginning on a preset date to achieve a certain weight loss and specific fitness level increase or decrease the effectiveness of the desired results?

Accordingly, the action plan is in place. The list to follow is outlined and schedules are set.

Here we go . . .

So on day one, we've got this. We're really going to make it happen this time. We've laid out a full calendar to get fit this year and have our first week's workout schedule. Monday morning we wake up early to go for a run through the neighborhood, then have time to come back and shower before leaving for work. We're so excited. We can't wait to get the process started. After work, we're going to the new gym we just joined for a weight session with a friend and we are going to focus on upper body exercises. We used to do all of this, so we think it should be pretty simple to pick back up. We meet up at the gym with our newly purchased fitness attire looking good and feeling good—stretch, lift those weights, cool down, and grab a towel. That was awesome. We really missed this. There was a little newness to it all as we looked around the place to make sure we knew what we were doing and basically fit in with the overall surroundings. Some of the equipment looked different, but we were able to figure it all out. All done, and we feel great with day one in the books. We did it!

Day two, we're cycling on the new stationary bike we just got. We get a workout in before showering. Then after work, we're focusing on the lower body and we're still feeling good with day two in the books. We did it again!

Day three, we wake up early and run again. And after work, we're back to some more upper body weights.

Day four is similar to day two with a few adjustments to change it up. We are definitely feeling it today. A little sore and achy, but that was expected.

Day five is an alternate day, working on all of those little muscles and different areas of concentration that we sometimes don't get to in the major muscle groups. We add in some yoga and relaxation techniques with a local yoga class held by the river and are feeling great. It's absolutely gorgeous outside and we are full of inspiration.

Then we use the weekend to go for a light walk and recover the body so we're fresh and ready to go again on Monday for week two—still feeling good.

We make it to Monday of the third week of January by doing pretty much the same sorts of routines and commitments and, so far, we're on track to be more fit and healthy this year. But then Wednesday hits, and Wednesday is hump day of course and boy did we wake up tired, rolling out of bed with a deep breath or two and a shrug . . . this isn't going to be fun this morning, and it's cold and wet outside anyway. Maybe we'll get a few more winks . . . and then time has run out. We will just make the workout up at lunch; however, we had to work through lunch with so much to do, so we'll just get the run in after work this evening. But then it's dark, and we're exhausted anyway.

And then, all of the sudden, it's Thursday and we get home from work and boy what a day it was. We're tired, but we still haven't done the things we committed to do at the beginning of January weeks ago. We tell ourselves it's okay, we'll double down tomorrow, get up a little earlier and stay up a little later and kinda sorta marry the two days and still get in all the stuff we had planned. But then it's Friday, and we're so glad it's Friday. What a week it's been. We're invited to go to dinner and still haven't gotten to our list yet, but that's okay, the weekend is coming, and we have plenty of time Saturday to get all of this stuff caught up and back on track.

In the blink of an eye, it's Sunday evening, and we're still buried under our list and it's been bugging us all weekend. In fact, we're trying to get it out of our mind, because it's kind of bringing us down a little.

It's now Monday, the fourth week of January, and we're so far behind on our plans for this year that we're a little deflated and constantly thinking about how hard this is going to be for another eleven months after not even making it through a single month yet.

So it goes with millions of people every year—this continual cycle, this roller coaster of excitement toward the 'new me.'

Who said that you would be ready on December 31 anyway? Who came up with this idea that the new year had to equal a new you? It's truly not how humans are wired.

Of course, we do have triggers in our life that make us decide to do something. We make up our minds to go for our dreams, or capture our inner strength, etc. Sometimes monumental events snap us to do something, make this change or that, to get a thing done or make a commitment that lasts a lifetime. But that's a gamble I'm not going to bet on. Needing some twist of fate, good or bad, welcoming or painful, exciting or desperate to make me accomplish my dreams, goals or to pursue a passion with complete confidence over a certain period is not for me.

What we really want is to be in complete control of the entire process. We want to make our decisions and act on them with assured strength.

For sure New Year's will bring the question: What do I want to accomplish in the coming year? And I do think setting goals for the upcoming year (or the identified period) is important. What I've come to do is start by taking an account of the last important period, whether that's a year or a chapter of my life, and I work to determine what went right and what went wrong. Once I have a good understanding of those factors. I can begin figuring out what to do better, ways to improve on what was successful and avoid the things that weren't.

So, I set my new resolutions, whether or not I end up verbalizing them, write them down, sharing them with someone close to me, or keeping them to myself. I set my goals with an action plan and dates of achievement to keep me on track past the second week. For example, on July 1, I begin directing my thoughts and feelings toward the second half of the year and what it might bring. It's the time to fulfill and complete what I started in the first half of the year. To run toward the finish line, so to speak, and finish the race with a robust effort.

If I've learned anything on this journey of life, of setting resolutions and learning to keep them, it's that I have to keep going, traveling toward the destination that will unearth the answers my soul so deeply desires to find.

They say that youth is wasted on the young, but I won't accept that. That cannot be the way it was meant to be. Something is telling me that I am called to do more, which may, in fact, mean doing less.

We are all so different, yet we have so many similarities. Everyone has a heart that beats, blood that runs through their veins, skin and cells that die and recreate themselves continually. We all have a brain that can think and learn and decide, arms and legs to help us through the tasks of the day, eyes that are made to give sight. Yet, the effects of life on the body seem to be so drastically different for everyone. The dating of bodies, minds, organs, and even wills tends to be so very different. So, once again I wonder: How much control do I have on those effects, or is it out of my control completely? Is it just a matter of randomness?

I must know the answers to these questions, so I will continue to forge on this quest, continue to climb the volcano that's been here since the earliest civilization. As this ancient civilization was developing—and thriving—what did they know? What did they understand and learn about themselves that allowed them to thrive as they did? Was it instinctual? Was it experiential? I simply had to know more.

Modern-day culture and civilization owe a lot to these earliest civilizations. Our civilization had come a long way from an age when there were no defined means of communication and hunting was the primary source of food. Gradually, foraging evolved into agriculture, animals were domesticated, societies were created and developed, and we eventually reached the societies we live in today. Each individual civilization contributed new inventions, new ideas, new cultures, philosophies, lifestyles, etc. From the very cradle of civilization, what we have become is a result of all civilizations that came before.

The purpose of this journey to the volcano was to find guidance from 10,000 years ago, from this particular cradle of civilization, that might point me toward my next destination and clearer answers. If there was a message thus far, my theory was that it would be about the constancy of practice at the most rudimentary place. But getting to that rudimentary place would be challenging for me. I had created a life full of intense organizational patterns, schedules, goals, and plans that filled each and every day. In fact, I was usually scheduled hour by hour throughout the day, and my checklist of accomplishments, which was very long, was becoming confusion and clutter, check marks and scratched-out lines on the pages. Setting a particular date for resolutions was really not that effective in most cases. And for a lifelong goal setter, with progress identifiers, expectations, and completion dates, this didn't sit very well.

So, to set aside my pattern of goal setting with timelines in clinical columns was going to be just a little bit of a challenge.

That's why after studying the simple lives of these ancient Mesoamericans, I believed they may have understood a way of life that eludes us today with our super sophisticated, complex lifestyles. My new understanding of achieving a goal was to take a desire and break it down to the simplest form that I could construct in my mind and begin practicing it regularly without ever missing one period. That's it. Preferably this was something that could be so simple, so easy, that it would take little to no energy; however, the one thing that was not negotiable was rehearsing it consistently for my designated daily period. In fact, even the time spent rehearsing relative to the time of day could be flexible, so that when life events adjusted my timeframe without warning, the scheduled exercise would simply continue at a different time that day.

Ultimately, the rehearsal would obtain the desired result, and it would become part of me and my lifestyle conditioning, an enhanced enjoyment fulfilling other parts of my life. My study and historical trip down the Mesoamerican trail to the volcano brought me to that place. And so I found myself traversing a volcanic mountainside to seek the next clue that would shed some light on my path ahead, on this new way of achieving key objectives and formulating patterns.

Not surprisingly, this was a first for me. Sliding down the inside of a volcano was not something I ever thought I would do, nor something I would have considered advisable or perhaps even possible. Nevertheless, there I was, sliding down the inside of this extraordinary volcano embracing all of its ancient secrets.

I don't know why, but I thought that it would be dead, dry, and crusty. I thought it would be quite a hard surface, but it wasn't. It was more like walking in a mountain range. There was even some vegetation and other signs of life as time and nature perform their magic. And it wasn't hot or even warm as one might imagine but quite cool, which was probably a really good sign. The particular volcano I was climbing had not been active for some time, more than a hundred years to be accurate, so I was feeling fairly confident that I was not going to be cooked alive.

Another interesting part is that the volcano was not just straight down, like a cone in science or chemistry class. When I decided to do this climb, I conducted some research and made sure that the inside of these dormant volcanoes, basically a giant mountainous cave formed by congelation of lava or accumulation of volcanic breccia, was going to be manageable to walk and maneuver until I reached the level where I might be able to reach these stone structures that held critical pieces of information for my journey to continue. However, these expectations were all in theory prior to actually arriving on the scene so, as usual, some faith would be required.

Once I had descended approximately 150 meters into this beast of a volcano, all visibility from natural light dissipated, and it was just me and my trusty lighting gear. I was nearing the depth the map indicated, hoping for some sign that I was in the right place. After a few more meters, to my wonderment, I saw it—a landing of some sort.

Well, I'm being a little generous by calling it a landing. It was more of a rugged, sharp-edged configuration jutting from the side of this volcano's belly. As I drew closer, I could make out, barely, what was likely to be the artifacts my trusted counselors, safely back at their residential seclusions, and I were hoping to find. They looked like structures that could have been made by someone, but they could also have been big rocks breaking away from the inside layer of the volcano from years of natural wear, decay, and settlement.

I looked at my drawings (like a child reading a book with a flashlight under the covers after lights out), and back up again at the stones. Again and again, I repeated that process. Stepping a little closer, something caught my eye. There, not right in front of me, but as I worked my way around the edge of this landing, again, a term loosely used, a form began to distinguish itself from the rock wall.

As I continued to move gently to the left, the shape became clearer.

Lo and behold, it was, without question, a carved structure. In fact, there were four of them clear as day. Mind you, I was standing on a ledge that I wasn't completely sure was stable to get a clear view. But it was exactly as described in the drawings and the research from my advisors.

I took a moment to gather and secure myself on this ledge and coordinate with my surroundings before I more closely examined these beauties. Believing that I was safely stabilized, I began gathering all of the data and imagery I could. There was writing as well as artwork on each of the stones. I adjusted the lights and got several angles, drawing in detail as best I could under the conditions. I worked diligently to preserve every facet of the scenes, which I thought must not have been touched—or even seen—in hundreds of years. Once sufficiently satisfied with the success of my documenting, I began my ascent, which was no easy task. It's much simpler to get inside of a volcano than to climb back out.

Once I was out in the light again safely, standing on top of the volcano, I took a moment to contemplate what I had just experienced and what all of it must mean. Was this the secret I had been looking for? Was it a series of clues? Or was it a guide to the next stop on my discovery voyage?

All I knew was that I could not wait to get back to the institute for some assistance deciphering and organizing all of this data in order to formulate its meaning . . . and decide where my next stop would be.

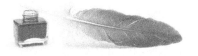

Chapter 4

MIND GAMES

THE INDUS VALLEY CIVILIZATION

I walked up to the very edge, or at least the best I could decipher to be the edge considering the vastness of the plateau. The terrain overwhelmed the senses, reaching over 1,000 kilometers from the eastern lands to the western boundary. It is the greatest highland in all the world, stretching some 2,500,000 kilometers in total. The average elevation is over 4,500 meters and the mountain range holds Mount Everest and K2 (the Savage Mountain as it is sometimes referred) in its palm, the highest summits on the planet.

This mesa is often considered the 'roof of the world.' There are many ways to move about; however, just going from one point to another leaves little room for really experiencing it. Accordingly, I chose to travel by horse through the region, along the ancient riverbeds, in order to get a greater understanding of where I am in this massive landscape. With such a wondering mind, I have found that the serenity of a space gives me peace and calm. It's in that kind of serene space that I discovered so much more about who I am—or hope I am—and who I hope I can become.

This amazingly beautiful land was the gathering and filtering source for all of the region's water supply, known as the water tower with its thousands of ice glaciers, maintaining the rivers and streams that serve the massive landscape in its wake. The freshwater reserve contains the shelf for the grandest ice fields on the planet other than those in the polar regions, thus its nickname of 'the Third Pole.'

Even though this journey would take some time, I was jubilant to be on it. It may have been the most free I had ever felt in my entire life. I could go in any direction, having not really allotted a specific time to get to the plateau. I was anxious to reach it; however, I didn't want to miss anything along the way. So, it was on purpose that I traveled slowly and lived inside of the consciousness I had adapted in the days leading up to landing at this wondrous place amid the Tibetan Plateau. For a few weeks, I rode and walked and camped among the stars. I read and wrote and listened to whatever I needed to. Along the way, I saw nature everywhere, the eternal cycle of life all around me.

By the eighth day, I was a little blistered and sore, to be honest, but that was to be expected. Although the land was glorious and beautiful, it was also pure nature and could be unforgiving, as I assumed it had been since the beginning of time. Most importantly though, I had come upon a Himalayan marmot, exceedingly natural to this terrain which told me I was on the right path, getting closer to reaching the landing site where I would begin the ascent.

I wondered what the marmot was thinking . . . I suppose it was probably just making its way through life, doing what it does, not thinking of much else. Of course, many things in life are a mystery, but isn't that the point? To search for those mysteries, to live with an earnest excitement for each moment?

I know it's not easy, but living in search of life's mysteries is certainly worth pursuing with every bone in one's body. Where does that come from anyway? That desire to pursue something, anything. Why is it that the human spirit alone strives so desperately to find their desired way?

I've always had that desire—always, of that I'm certain—but for what . . . I've never been quite as sure. Hence, the desire to find the 'what' that drives me and, for that matter, anyone. I would run—or stumble—down this path and that one, and then another. I was never aimlessly wandering. It always seemed like my purpose was a focused result, no matter what the result was; however, sometimes I felt a little lost or confused during each goal pursued, wondering what was driving me, why I was pursuing this thing.

Looking back now, I believe that was the journey I had to take in order to find my way. There is a strength that only comes from doing. It doesn't matter that someone else may have done it and shared their point of view; it is something you must experience on your own.

I think that may be part of the beauty that I've discovered. Eventually, the paths start to align themselves in a meaningful way. There is a confidence that comes from having put them together, like pieces of a puzzle that only I could shape. And not just the puzzle, but the shapes they outline, the number of pieces, the size of the puzzle pieces, the colors, thickness, and texture. Now I see that it's my puzzle—mine alone. It, of course, has had lots of influences along the way from the special people in my life and all of the other associations that direct my decision-making process, but in the end, it is mine alone.

Isn't it amazing, when you look back at the line of your life, how it is simpler than it looked while in the midst of developing? No matter how difficult it seemed during those developmental times, it becomes palatable. I certainly don't want to repeat some experiences, and hopefully, I won't have to, but just knowing that I can make it through the things I have gives me an element of belief in my own ability to climb the next mountain and reach that next plateau—quite literally, in my case.

Just think about when you had a troubling concern that wouldn't allow your mind to rest. No matter what you tried to do to create other distractions and free your mind from this ornery pest, it just kept presenting itself in vivid, unrelenting manners in an effort to control your mind space. It just moved in and took up a room as if to say 'I'm here and I'm not going anywhere.' Most fascinating is when you make it past that one pesky concern and, looking back later, it isn't as prevalent. This one thing that owned your mind for a period with unusual domination, is now, although still recallable, fuzzy at best and over time gets even more blurry.

This all brought me to the conclusion, that, yes, as the saying goes, this too shall come to pass. The next morning arrives and I find I'm still here. The new day has dawned, the sun has risen, and I'm alive.

So, if we know that's the case, why do we spend so much time, energy, effort, stress, emotion, thought, and fret over this thing? Why do we allow our minds to be manipulated so easily and fully by this gnat?

Now, I know you might say that I don't understand, that what you're dealing with is real and serious and life-changing and scary and too much to handle. I get it, and I'm not downplaying the truly mind-blowing experiences in this thing we call life. Some things are nearly, well, actually, completely impossible for the human brain and heart to grasp. Things that make us ask: How could this happen to me? Or to that innocent soul? How does something like that take place in our world? Why does God allow such a thing? I understand and have always believed that there is an event that will require obedience even to the strongest foe. However, the overwhelming majority of things fit into the prior category: they just aren't that big of a deal. It only *seems* they are due to our station in life, or where our relative maturity and understanding are at the time when this challenge raises its trying head.

When I come across a challenge, I have always believed that I will just overcome it. Just go for it. Work harder. Set my goals, put my action plan in place, and achieve the end result. But with a number of years and case studies to prove that was not the case, my belief system started to change. Yes, I still believe in all of the positive elements of life, and I know how important it is to stay the course toward your desired outcome, but I also believe that staying the course with blinders on alone is how many fail to achieve the results they hoped for.

After many years of experimental cycles, I came to believe that the mind is the last thing to arrive when you are pursuing a goal.

In fact, your mind will likely get in the way and slow you down on your journey—and that's the good news. If the mind is what usually gets in the way of me achieving my dreams, why do so many people want to believe that the mind is the key element to overcoming challenges or getting to their goal?

That's right, I decided I needed to get my mind out of my way.

Not that the mind is not a wonderful blessing and tool, but it can only be a tool if it has been trained as such.

And there's the tricky part.

It's a 'what goes in is what comes out' scenario. Well, not exactly like that, but I wish it were that easy to explain. Training the mind is more of a long-term conditioning process for this special muscle in order for it to perform for greater control, success, fulfillment, joy, happiness, accomplishment, recognition, and so much more.

Let me try explaining another way. The world might say . . .

Just do it.
Go for it.
Find your inner strength.
Make a decision.
Never give up.
Greatness takes time.
Be patient.
Courage is one step ahead of fear.
Focus on your goal.
Always look toward your dream.
The only person you will become is the person you decide to be.

Don't get me wrong. I love all of these expressions and yearn to live by them each and every day; however, it has proven to be very difficult for humans to stay on track for any meaningful period of time when they depend on their mind alone. This thing happens and then the next thing happens, all disrupting the well-intended plan.

I had a friend who once told me they wanted to really improve their eating habits, become more nutritionally aware, and live a healthier life. Every once in a while, I would ask how that was going, to which they would respond, "I was doing really well and losing weight, I felt better, I had more energy and excitement about life, then I went on this trip and it just threw me back into my old habits again and I'm back to where I was before I started."

This has also happened to me many, many times over. I was committed. I believed. I made the effort . . . and then I took a trip, or I had a bad day, or I had an interruption of one kind or another and was back to the starting blocks all over again. That's ultimately just frustrating, so I would throw up my hands and give up, thinking that one day maybe I would actually figure out how to stay on track, how to control the mind and have enough willpower to achieve my goals.

Truthfully, I think it's human nature to believe that we're in control. We think we're strong and can handle anything. Perhaps that's how our minds have been trained. I know mine was trained that way. I was always vehemently determined to accomplish a feat, no matter how long it took, no matter the cost.

Learning that didn't work was a difficult lesson for me, and it took a long time for me to accept, whether that was from stubbornness, pride, fear, or something else.

I would start with incredibly high levels of motivation. Passion is a beautiful thing, and I love it. And then I would research. There are literally thousands, if not millions, of articles, books, podcasts, websites, experts, teachers, trainers, specialists, gurus, coaches, and facilities that will blow your mind and offer all sorts of advice for whatever you're trying to achieve. They tell you to do this or don't do that (and of course, not all of them agree). But I would sort through the information and think: I can do that! I've got this! This is going to be so easy.

All of this focus and innovation is awesome, but the more study I completed, the more research I participated in, and the more case studies I examined, the more I started to see what I was doing wrong. Then instead of trying to figure out how I could conquer my mind and force it to focus, the realization came that I was requesting the wrong action from this particular muscle, and the goal became figuring out how I could get my mind out of my way and, more specifically, train it. It has a much more illustrious purpose, and this was not it.

This amazing muscle we call the brain is, without question, the most fascinating creature of our existence save the soul (which is a completely different and even deeper conversation). However, its understanding and examination leaves one in endless bouts of illusions, fascinations, highs, and lows . . . enough to transcend civilizations, galaxies, and, for that matter, universes.

For example, I can know something absolutely, with confidence and surety of my next move, and seconds later a faulty foundation full of questions and uncertainty throws me into a tailspin.

So how do you get in control of this thing? The mind is like an alien with its own life and direction. It has a personalized map and a plan for the day, minute by minute . . . but it's mine. I should be in control of my own mind, shouldn't I? But what does that even mean?

Who leads who anyway? Is the brain this autonomous decision-maker? Does it operate on its own, or does the human in which it resides decide to go left or right, up or down? Many times, I am not sure . . . we tell the brain what we want it to think, right? We want to go in this direction, slightly to the right, or around the corner to the left.

Or does the independent muscle tell its host what to do and we respond by bumping into things, getting bruised and cut, sore and smarting until we figure it out?

As I continued thinking through all of this, I really didn't know what to do with my mind—but I wanted to find out, whatever it took.

As I understand it, some 40,000 thoughts run through our minds each day and 85 percent of those are negative. Who made those odds? That's not fair or even reasonable. I at least wanted a 50 percent shot at gaining control of this giant residing above my shoulders.

On the other, more positive hand, this thing is capable of amazing feats that stun the most enthusiastic adventurer, lifting them up beyond the stars, or dropping them to their knees in total submission.

Sometimes it is a simple episode that moves the thoughts racing and wandering. In other cases, it is huge, even breathtaking to witness. Things that make you wonder if they are even possible. Occurrences that are superhuman and out of this world. How does a person climb up the face of an almost-flat mountain without a lifeline anchoring them to safety? Even though the human mind has such amazing capacity, I've always said not to tempt fate. There is something for every person that can bring them to their knees, no matter how on top of the world, accomplished, in charge, or secure they may believe their stance in life.

So, if this magnificent machine is so capable of both good and not-so-good, what is the steering mechanism? What guides the road on which it turns and the process by which it is directed? Does it even have one?

Let's assume that it does for a moment.

Let's assume the mind has a guidance system that stipulates the direction it is going to go. What is it? Could I be in charge of it? Could I tell it to climb this mountain and up it goes, without hesitation or restriction?

In fact, the mind is so pure that it doesn't believe it can be stopped, so powerful that it can achieve any task it is presented with. And at the same time it is limitless to achieve, it is also limitless in its ability to do harm or limit the desires of the body. It can just as easily make you depressed, or enter a state of insignificance, or feel unsuccessful in your life pursuits, unaccomplished, without joy, happiness, or completeness. I know, that's not much fun to think about, but it's oh so necessary.

If I am to defeat my challenger (the mind), I have to first understand it.

If I am going to lift myself up and overcome the challenges the universe presents, I must be ever-present and engaged with the enemy aspect of the mind, which is certainly real. I must be ever-present in the same way as I would be in the absolute presence of glory and beauty, greatness and wondrousness.

As I was there among the mountains.

There was a particular wonder that early night. The temperature was frigid and only survivable by the most ardent Tibetan warrior—or a properly geared visitor as I was.

I was completely sober in thought, adjusted to the surroundings after weeks in this special place, a world unto itself. A cup of very hot coffee helped to warm my insides as I stared off into the snow-laden mountainside, the light still present, gleaming off the white-faced cliffs of the steepest part of the climb remaining, so glorious, waiting to offer the challenge. As I drifted off into an utter completeness, I was startled by something nearby. I proclaimed my presence, asking if someone was there, catching a glimpse of movement perhaps one hundred meters straight above me, hanging off of the mountainside.

I blinked hard to make sure I wasn't hallucinating. In an attempt to adjust my sight and identify the outline above me, I stood at the base of this next crevasse, and I saw long hair, a strong and muscular outline gleaming down on me. It was a gorgeous sight to behold.

As if on cue, the dropping sun shone a bright light directly on the creature, making it appear to be on stage, performing for me alone. I had heard many stories of Yeti, or the elusive 'Big Foot,' but this was real, and it was right on top of me.

Of course, I didn't move, still not sure what it was or if it was human. With the natural spotlight providing a full view, and the creature looking directly down on me, with the only movement of either party being the smoke from my coffee and our breath in the cold air, the picture became clearer. It was not a human, although it could be mistaken for one easily standing upright and full-faced. Oh, that face! Pristine, full of confidence, as a ruler and sovereign of his land. Simply magnificent! It was blue while mine was red and chapped at best from the relentless cold, but the blue was not blue from the cold.

I began to recognize him, with his golden mane and snubbed nose. The infamous blue-faced Chinese monkey here in the Tibetan mountain wilderness. Now I know I'm square in the middle of my designed journey line. He was an old-world monkey, adjusted to this temperate mountain forest, at minus five degrees Celsius and 670 meters above sea level, where I was viewing this spectacular scene.

Looking down on me from its mountain throne, it appeared to be quite large; however, I had some knowledge of the animal life in this region. There are twenty-nine mammal species in Tibet, all of which are adapted to the country's low temperatures and high elevation. Accordingly, my recollection was that the monkey was more likely about one meter in height and forty kilos in weight. Nonetheless, it was a daunting sight, him being covered with lean, powerful muscles, a gorgeous orange fur coat, and that undeniable blue face, full of grace and majestic awe. The orange and tan tail was almost as long as the creature is tall.

With only some 10,000 or so remaining on the entire planet, this encounter was all the more magnificent. It's one thing to be on an expedition to discover one of these fabulous beings, but a chance encounter on the frozen side of the mountain at dusk had to mean something more.

I hadn't seen anyone for days, so even though I was taken aback and, admittedly, a little frightened (not that he needed me for dinner, being a herbivore, but that he might have felt threatened or territorial, needing to defend himself or his roaming grounds), I tried to assure him that I meant no harm. I hoped he instinctively got it because he could have climbed down and taken me out in a matter of seconds if he had wanted to.

No doubt he was frightening, but he was breathtaking as well. Traveling alone, the monkey was likely a male, even though the species does live communally with several females and their babies. He most likely was just doing what he does, finding his way, providing a life as complete and natural and free as any creature could ever hope.

I took some comfort that he appeared not to be that interested in me and slowly began to calm down and enjoy witnessing his remarkable favor and beauty as he went about his way, marching through the thick, snowy carpet to his next destination. Surely, he must have been heading home to the sanctuary of his habitat and, perhaps, family after a full day of exploration.

Reflecting on the experience, my mouth curled into a slight grin, knowing that we were fairly similar, going about our missions toward some end, wondering if maybe it was simpler for him. Does he fret over things that really don't matter much, or does he consistently stay enamored with only the truly important aspects of his day, continuously living in the present? That would be a grand feat for anyone, as it's nearly unobtainable for humankind; yet, perhaps it is normal for other creatures on this earth.

While I spent the next few minutes wondering, my fascinating, blue-faced friend decided it was time to move along, and, with the swiftness and deliberateness of something superhuman, he climbed the snow-covered face of the mountain as if it were an afternoon stroll down a slight hill.

Watching him go, I was inspired and decided that I would go ahead and continue my climb. After many hours, I finally arrived and leaped over the top.

As I was standing on the roof of the world, the plateau below revealed its vastness and remained a daunting sight, but the toughest part of my journey was behind me. I continued along the path I had mapped in a labor of love. This place was massive, wild and grand in all its glory. Diligence in effort would be required to get to my destination.

Following my days of riding and hiking, I arrived at what I believed to be the right place. The goal in this Indus Valley wilderness was to locate the Indus Script sites, or Harappan script as they are also called, Harappan being the model of an archaeological culture, an identification technique relating to its archeological excavation that began in the early twentieth century.

It was the first site of its kind to come from these ancient Indus civilizations being revealed, and its actual discovery took place during the British Raj by the Archeological Survey of India. The script sites contained a corpus with symbols and inscriptions, most of which were very short, and it was difficult to determine if they were a language or some type of writing system, making them all the more intriguing to the researcher as they seemed to throw most normal linguistic syntax, rules, processes, and principles out the window. To complicate it further, the symbols would vary by location.

I got down on the ground and crawled around to review the surroundings and far beneath the site, there it was. Lying undiscovered were hundreds of pieces of broken tablets, all small and ridged and in no special order. Secretly hidden beyond the Indus Script discovery as it stands was a pathway to a long, dark, thin, rough hall that led to these pieces of broken script. I had to duck down when the hall declined in height. It was claustrophobic at minimum, wet, and dark.

I had a little light from my equipment, and from the looks of the surroundings, no one had been there for thousands of years, maybe never since its original creation. The Indus Script as it stood was discovered more than a century ago, but its meaning or intent had not been deciphered since the language, if that's what it was, had no comparable dialect to date.

In an effort to make sure the inscriptions I found were of a different kind than the current archives of the Indus Script collection, I combed through all of the known research available from my shorthand reference notes. Of course, much more extensive examination would be required once I had transported them back to the institute and the established research consortiums. You see, the additional transcripts could have been some of the most significant in the Far East and Mediterranean complex if they proved to be worthy. Considering the significance, the safekeeping of these artifacts was utterly essential.

Feeling confident that mine was a unique discovery of new Indus Script elements, I returned to the institute for assistance in determining the relevance of the tablets. Even though others had uncovered certain traces of the Indus Script, this particular text appeared never to have been seen before.

Back at the institute, a history lesson ensued regarding writing on stone, rock, or cave walls during the Stone Age. One of the researchers told me the common writings of the Ancient Greeks were in stone, a form known as boustrophedon. This writing style is described as a bi-directional text, mostly inscriptions and engravings. The line directions alternate, going from left to right and then right to left in opposition to European languages, which go left to right, and the Arabic or Hebrew languages that go right to left. Additionally, the letters or characters are reversed; it takes a mirror to put them in the correct viewing order.

After thoroughly reviewing the stone etchings, one particular historian erupted with a yelp and then didn't stop. He was yelling and cheering; his ramblings were in a language foreign to me. He was running around the room like a child chasing a friend through a field. I stayed out of the way, mainly because I didn't know him very well, but I also didn't want to get trampled, and I didn't know what to expect next. So, I kept a safe distance in the corner of his laboratory, attempting to meld into the bookshelves and remain out of view.

Eventually, he came to a stop, slowly bent over, placed his hands on his knees, and dropped his head toward the floor. I was still hiding, waiting with bated breath.

After what seemed to be several minutes, but was probably only seconds, he raised his head, looked right at me (so much for the blending in), and asked, "Do you know what this is?"

"No," I said.

Inside my head, I said: Of course I don't know, that's why I brought it to you.

"You have uncovered what archeologists, researchers, historians, and scientists have been desperately pursuing for decades. You see, we have the script—the Indus Script—in many forms from many sites, yet no one has been able to unlock what it says. There are lots of theories and opinions but no agreement on any of them . . .but that's all about to change my friend.

"You have discovered the cipher," he continued. "This code is the key to not only reading the Indus Script but to locating the hidden writings of the Indus Valley peoples."

I had yet to share with him that I had, in fact, discovered the additional transcripts as I examined the entire cave system after finding what I now understood to be the key cipher. Fortunately, I had brought the other manuscripts that I found in the same cave system as the cipher. Excited to move on to the accompanying manuscripts and their meaning, the researcher informed me that it would take some time to organize and catalog the cipher in an orchestrated algorithm to identify and apply it to multiple languages. In fact, he informed me that it would take several weeks at a minimum.

A little frustrated after receiving that news, I needed to regain perspective on where my journey was headed—and what was at stake. As I sat in the lobby of my hotel after a long trip back to Wuhan and the institute, I contemplated what to do next. It became abundantly clear that I needed to forge ahead since I wouldn't be of much value to the tedious deciphering process.

The next stage of the journey, although ultimately related, could be independently pursued, and since I was already in China, I began making the necessary arrangements immediately.

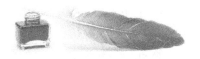

Chapter 5

THE CASCADE

HEAVEN LAKE, CHINA

This place is so remote. Returning to China, it was utterly breathtaking. To think that this journey had taken me all over the world to reveal such amazing, yet simple, explanations of how and why humans are here on this planet. I was so close to where I needed to be the whole time . . . to only find my way there late in the journey seemed appropriate considering what a trek it had been.

Looking back, I'm not sure it could have been any other way. It may not have been possible to get there without going through the other corridors first or, for that matter, in the specific order in which they were presented.

As the helicopter flew toward the mountain range and crater, we climbed higher and higher, cresting more than 2,000 meters in elevation at the top of the snow-capped mountain range.

Atop the white steeples, experiencing a rush so full that everything seemed to move in slow motion, I could see and hear everything with unbridled clarity. All of my senses were performing at an extremely elevated level. The wind was blowing the loose snow from the caps, and I could count each flake individually, hear the sound of the helicopter blades whirling at the controlled beat of a bass drum, whipping every four count. The birds flying over the horizon seemed to be gliding, their wings flittering up and down as if to pause between each flap.

As we cleared the mountain peaks, the water came into view for the first time. What a wondrous sight to see. It was clear why this venue received its name: Heaven Lake. It was heavenly, to be sure. In ancient Chinese literature, it was called Tianchi or Nanming, which translates to 'southern sea.' Without question, it was the most spectacular view I had ever seen, and I had been all across this miraculous planet.

The water is crystal blue, so clear I could practically see the bottom some 381 meters deep, looking like a fishbowl in which you could see every ounce of water. From the angle we were coming in, the entire mountain surrounding the crater and the lake itself appeared to nestle comfortably among the clouds. Off in the distance, I could see the landscape shooting in and out between the rising and dipping peaks, with a rainbow of colors as far as the eye could see.

I had just come back to earth as the pilot began his gradual descent into one of the crevices we had outlined in our operational meetings a few days prior. He was a true professional. Having never seen this sight before either, he still managed to perform the smoothest of landings. Settling down in the picturesque canvas, we were right on schedule.

Stepping onto the ground for the first time was surreal, as it felt somewhat weightless. I knew we were still on earth, but it just felt like gravity was less present there. No one was floating away, but this place was unsurpassed in beauty and solitary in expression. Gathering the simplest of packs and equipment for the hike and climb ahead, there was a reverence expected. Not a word was spoken. It was just natural, like I was supposed to be there. This place was expecting my arrival, and it was saying: Welcome home.

It was interesting that the further back my travels took me, the simpler things became, and the closer to the beginning of living I transcended. The simplicity of those beginnings—those first ancient civilizations—have revealed themselves through the scribes recorded by the ancient city of Wuhan and the region's Chinese tribes.

And that brings me to another thought: Humanity, as wonderful as it is, with its unbelievably beautiful spirit, still finds it very difficult to accept these simple principles that have been uncovered. These principles that have been actually received without resistance, these truths that are, in fact, real, pure, and exact.

It's probably not a surprise to most people that societies tend to complicate many elements of daily living, which could be for many reasons. Perhaps one is the disbelief that life could be so simple. Another could be a conditioned belief that a process must work because that's the way it's always been done. People express this opinion and that opinion, which leads to this solution and then another. Then come the many rules that continue to complicate what was naturally designed to be simple and straightforward.

There is also the intelligence ego, which can capture us all from time to time. We think there's no way something can be that simple, so we're going to figure it out on our own. We don't want our intelligence insulted by being told that we should follow a very simple, almost childlike, naive path. We think we will arrive at the answer on our own, and we're not buying the simplicity. We keep going down our own path, thinking we'll keep driving ahead until we reach our goal. We know we're right, and we aim to prove it.

I myself continued to pursue the journey in order to understand the dream, this dream that was so elusive for me. I was within maybe an hour of that very site in China so many times. But it felt as if I were on another planet when I finally went.

How did I get there anyway?

(After a while, all the travels begin to run together.)

In some ways, it was wonderful, because there are no concerns when you are across the world far from any other human being.

But after a few days, it is easy to start missing the human connection as well. I began thinking about all the people who mean so much to me. What were they doing right that minute? Where were they, and what were they thinking about?

It was nice to see all of that beauty and feel free, yet yearn for those who are so important to me and have had a significant impact on my life. It was an interesting dichotomy, but both sentiments were good, I think.

That place . . . I had never seen anything like it before. I followed the instructions provided in the brief to the letter, but I wasn't expecting anything that amazing, and I was wondering how it stayed a secret for so long. How is there not a resort right in the middle of where I was standing? Was I still on earth, or had I been transported to another planet? I remember traveling all that distance, but it seemed so vague once I was looking at Heaven Lake.

I was confident that I had not been drugged, and I was pretty sure I was awake and coherent during the entire journey . . . so why did I feel like I had entered another time zone or another galaxy in outer space?

My dear friend once told me that if I wanted to connect with someone I love, I needed to look into their eyes. If I looked into their eyes, I would see their very soul, their true self, and the heart that will reveal their truest nature. And it's true, sometimes I have not really looked into someone's eyes and given them all of my attention in order to truly see them. There's a difference when you look into someone's eyes. My hope is that people can see others at their most wondrous in each moment, as I was seeing my journey in that place.

When I arrived on the continent, I knew it would be very different than so many of the other places I had traveled to; however, it really was reminiscent of a movie, a living, breathing fantasy. It almost felt like it wasn't real. Standing there, I still wasn't sure if I was awake or dreaming.

Getting to that point was not easy . . . but it should have been.

In fact, that was the very point I believe I'm being led to understand: the simplicity of our universe. Our existence was not meant to be so complicated. We did this to ourselves. Our societal ambitions create this desire to be different, to be better than the next person.

Please don't get me wrong, I believe in ambition and passion, the desire to achieve, and all of the elements of accomplishment that are attractive to so many millions around the world, but that's not the point. In this pursuit of accomplishment, sometimes I feel that we miss out on the opportunity to reach our ultimate potential, to actually be full. I've always thought of anything not on the path to the goal as a distraction, although most often it was just that I had difficulty recognizing it in its purest form. I think many things are distractions, and it is hard to keep our eye on the ball with so many bright, shiny lights everywhere.

Speaking of distractions, it was starting to get cold up at Heaven Lake, really cold. The temperature was dropping at a very rapid pace. I pulled out my parka, some gloves, and a head cap as a light but continual snow fell. It was the kind of breathtaking cold that overwhelms you. I've been a runner all my life, so I recognized that feeling of exuberance that you also get when you go for a run at a high altitude in a mountain town and the temperature is near freezing. I've always thought it to be an exhilarating feeling—full of life. Your lungs can breathe so deeply during the exertion and sometimes that lingers even after the experience for a period of time. There is an excess of air and oxygen. You could say it's spiritual or ultimately satisfying, a natural drug. If you've experienced it before, you know that feeling. Of course, the rush of endorphins, dopamine, and other neuromodulators adds to the state of exuberance too. Let's just say that the runner's high is actually a real thing, and I was experiencing the same feeling there.

It was unusual though because I was just standing there. There was no running happening. I had been in the same spot for about an hour, yet I was receiving that same feeling—the runner's high. That flood of endorphins coursing through my veins.

What was causing it?

The sun started to set, and the sky was a mysterious array of colors. It was more of the darker pallet of colors, yet it was also full of energy and life. A flowing, colorful work of abstract art. I believe mystical would be a fitting description.

As the darkness settled in, the sky continued to perform its symphony with brighter colors, like a rainbow following the rain, once the sun arrives back on the scene, with a full chorus as the light show danced across the vast open space of the heavens above.

I had traveled millions of kilometers in my lifetime, yet this was one show that I had never had the pleasure of watching. Certainly not anything like it.

I took a seat right there on the lake's snowy edge and enjoyed every single moment. It was like I had a reservation, and the actors were performing for me as the single invited guest, so I accepted the invitation and yielded with my undivided attention.

It was a glorious evening.

Since I had arrived back in China, I had been anxious to find this venue and see if it would actually lead me to this event. It wasn't the final stop—if there even is one—but I already knew it was part of the ultimate journey for me.

However, if all of the efforts and studies of so many idiomatic talented savants, separated by their individualistic pursuits, were now conjoined with a pursuit that is mine alone, I knew this would be the final revealing we were looking for to reach the journey's pinnacle.

After walking for several kilometers around the lake's edge, I was harnessed and anchored and all alone, lowering myself down to the bottom, or at least what I hoped was the bottom of this rugged, ribbed cavern. It was a silo cut into the base of the crevice around the lake's shore, almost impossible to find. As I descended, my visibility was extremely limited, but, remarkably, the temperature was relatively the same as the surface—without the falling snow, of course. The lower I got, the more gentle running water began to show up, sliding down parts of the walls around me.

Suddenly, a glimpse of reflection appeared as my eyes continued to adjust to the darkness, making me feel as if I was near the landing area beneath the cave shaft. I could see what appeared to be a rough rock landing below.

Grounded and unharnessed from my ropes and gear, I took a minute to gather my senses as I adjusted to my new environment. I was over-the-top nervous. It was a very small area, some oddly shaped space, with a narrow tunnel that led to an opening. I started walking in the only direction I could.

As I walked, still not comforted by the enclosure I had trapped myself in and feeling my way along the corridor, very faintly in the distance, a noise grew. It grew gently at first and then stronger, a static sound of sorts.

I wasn't sure what it was, so I continued to take soft, tip-toed, calculated steps toward the sound. I thought it might be water, running water, like a stream.

As I continued, it got louder and more distinct. It sounded more like rapids than a stream.

And louder and louder it drummed.

What was I walking into? It was thunderous at that point.

Whatever it was, I was holding onto the surrounding foundation as best I could, in expectation of a rush of water sweeping me away to nowhere. I knew I must be near an opening of some type, because it was now a full-flung production growing louder still, deafening and roaring.

I made it to the end of the cave walls that were clearly crafted by years of natural erosion from the elements. I reached for the edge of the tunnel with my left hand, slowly pulling myself through to see an underground pool system that was calm and stable; however, on the other side of the pool was a massive—and I mean massive—waterfall that lifted up toward the great cavern's peaks.

I couldn't hear myself yell, much less think. Not sure of the stability of the ledges around the large, naturally fueled pool, some thirty meters in circumference, I gingerly moved toward the waterfall to my right.

When I reached the waterfall, I turned on a powerful light system from my headgear to enhance the view of the tower castle, as I called it, of which I was a respectful guest at that point. As the light burst outward and upward in every direction, I was rewarded with the sight of a magnificently adorned place of lyrical wonder as the divine temple further exposed its beauty and serenity.

Then I noticed a slight opening at the back of the waterfall. It looked as if it might lead somewhere, so with an almost brazen perspective at this stage that came out of nowhere, I slid through the water's edge, getting trounced with falling walls of very thick cascading, powerful, confident layers of cold water. Instant loss of breath ensued from the experience.

Shaking off the excess water and brushing my hair back with my hand, gasping for air, trying to calm and regain composure, it hit me: Suddenly, there is no sound. It was completely quiet, still, and peaceful, as if I had made it backstage. I could still see some reflective light through the massive wall of water as I looked back toward the cave opening from behind the curtain. It was enough to provide a slight visual backdrop to the space I inhabited. With the additional light from my headgear, I could generally make out the area.

The shrine room, as I'm referring to it, was like a sphere. The edges were perfectly smooth, unlike those present throughout the rest of the cave system. It was reverent, like a small chapel more than one hundred meters below the lake's surface, toward the center of the lake.

And I had to wonder: What took place here?

Whether it was carved by nature, man, or some other force was unclear. Its purpose was equally unclear at that point, but I recorded everything I could see in multiple forms.

Then I moved closer and closer to examine the walled confines where I had found myself. Running my hands along the edges of the wall that had captured all of my attention, to my great surprise, I found a very tiny crease in the wall. I slipped my fingers and then my entire hand through without any backlash, and without any hesitation, miraculously, as if the space was growing, my entire body found its way following suit as well. I found myself behind the wall, which generated a sensation as if the walls were moving or rotating somehow to adjust and receive me on the other side; however, I could not make out any movement at all. It was my early assessment that one wall was offset just enough from the other wall's edge for me to slide between the stone's edges; regardless, once on the other side, the edges were completely gone. I could not see or feel the openings anymore, which caused some concern about eventually exiting the secret cave system I had wandered into. With the calling to move forward, I marked my location and continued believing there would be another way out when the time came.

After lifting myself around the wall's edge and looking upward, I was blessed with an unbelievable and overwhelming sight. There was *another* hidden cave. The space was over fifty meters in both height and width.

I had to just stop for a moment to take it all in.

In that instant, the reality set in that I was inside several inter-connected multi-cave systems, underneath a massive elevation, overwhelmingly beautiful lake, hundreds of meters below the surface of an area carved into the naturally formed mountains from an enormous crater impact some thousands of years in the making. It took few seconds to gather the full magnitude of this place—and perhaps the significance of the discovery in front of me.

Once I had become gathered again and established some stability emotionally, I surveyed my surroundings. At the other end of this massive hidden shrine room were several structures that I began to approach slowly. As I got closer, they grew, getting taller and taller. Once I was within twenty meters or so, the monolith pillars appeared to be as much as ten times taller than me. They were daunting, to say the least, impressive and audacious. I wasn't completely sure how I felt about them. All four of them seemed to signify an authority and spirituality that demanded reverence, and I was willing to oblige. If the obelisks were to provide ancient secrets, I was determined to deliver homage and receive their wisdom.

I retrieved as much information as I could, cataloging the angles, insignias, artistry, and carvings on the obelisks in exhausting detail. Although I was interested in the history and meaning behind those behemoth structures, I didn't want to underestimate their beauty or spiritual connection. They were breathtaking and glorious—to the point of inciting passion and, actually, a feeling of significance. In their presence, I began to get emotional. It was an ethereal sight to behold.

This hiding place beneath Heaven Lake had revealed all that one could imagine. Still consumed, I had completely forgotten about being in a stone enclosure without a way back out, but there was no expression of panic. Just as I had come through earlier, I looked back toward the monoliths again. The walls of granite were solid. This experience was a one-time affair. I would not be granted this sight ever again. After taking a moment to gain perspective, I started my ascent back to the surface. Regardless of the significance of the discovery, the experience was transformative, and it led to me becoming a different person from that point on.

Ultimately, the analysis of my finding would lead to us understanding that the access to the great truths revealed in Ancient Greece (the four pillars) was only attainable through a special process of submission and ownership. Finding ownership, and eventually becoming one with that ownership, was in and of itself a process that, although it was dramatically simple, would not be easy for us.

The multitude of caves and systems, journeys, trust, faith, confidence, and developed strength that came in time was, in fact, its own journey. In turn, it was only achieved if I were willing to take each and every step along the way. Reaching a plateau carved into this world would have forever evaded me, except that I submitted to the practice, which then led to the conditioning and, ultimately, ownership, allowing the next round of the process to occur. And each round led to greater and greater enlightenment of not life itself, but my own particular life.

Now that I had gained this knowledge, I found the strength that had always been right in front of me for so many years, just waiting for me to participate. See, that was the fascinating part. I was always trying too hard, wanting it too much. Believing some less-than-wise beliefs that it was a competition, or that something else was required, or that I needed a talent to allow me to gain this station in my own life. The clutter was so front-of-mind that not much else could be. But once I began to simply step back and became very good at the simplest of processes, the visionary openings became so clear. Some might think that this is an element of wisdom, but that wouldn't be accurate, as this is much deeper, broader, divine. More than philosophical, these attributes were encapsulated in and intertwined with the soul of man.

Here was the good stuff.

Each newly cascaded level of ownership came with a stronger ability to identify the next level of ownership, and each layer made it more simple, stronger, and clearer.

And so it went—over and over and over again.

This magnificent waterfall that carved mountains and formed a planet, fascinations, and fantasies happened simply, slowly, quietly . . . unnoticed at the beginning, but over time it became one of the most engaging, powerful, unstoppable wonders mankind has ever witnessed. The magnitude of this reality, now instilled in my brain, that *this* . . . yes, *this* might be the true cascading force that I was destined to unveil for all of humanity.

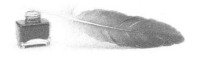

Chapter 6

THE FOUNTAIN

THE ISLAND OF BIMINI

I have always had a childlike faith. It's probably my greatest quality . . . always believing that something wonderful will happen.

Some might call that naive, but deep down, I always knew better.

I had a hope—a belief, actually—that I had a special reason for living, for being. That God had a plan specifically just for me.

I'm sure a lot of people feel that way. That there is a purpose only they can complete. A path only they can take on and fulfill. And as life teaches its lessons, those not always easily learned, that feeling becomes more concrete, whether they eventually find the purpose or not.

That feeling is not random.

Each one of us is here to do something—to help someone, to figure out why something is the way it is, to make a discovery, to find a solution, to reveal a truth. That purpose is different for everyone; however, I now know that each human's mission is to uncover the uniquely specific path that is laid out for them as an individual, a path that, quite frankly, no one else could, would, or should follow.

It's ours. Ours alone.

What a wondrous gift . . . to know that someone, somewhere has put us on our path since the beginning of time, since the instant the lights were turned on.

It has taken much of a lifetime (not that it really matters), but I now know for sure that this is mine. This is my path. My perfect line. So, when I finally reach my special destination, if I reach my special destination, I will stand in appreciation of that gift and be thankful for it, but I will be even more grateful for the passion granted to me in its pursuit. To be translucent is to allow transmitting or diffusing light so that objects cannot be seen clearly, as in water or a beauty seen beyond. This is where I had always found myself—in the lingering hope of eventually finding the ability, knowledge really, to gain access to the difficult-to-grasp, ultra-pure transparency.

One of the greatest illustrations throughout history has had many names and references. It denotes an elusive target, some attainment, or an objective of great significance. It has been described as the ultimate treasure, a subject matter of significant importance, especially in Arthurian literature. Some traditions have described it as a cup, a dish, or stone that possesses the power to grant joy, eternal youth, or sustenance in infinite abundance. It was first described as the vessel from which Jesus drank during The Last Supper, a vessel that Joseph of Arimathea would catch the blood of Christ at the Last Crucifixion of Christ, interlocking it for all time with the Holy Chalice.

The calling for my own personal attainment of significance was illuminated during all of my previous expeditions to the cradles of ancient civilizations and the subsequent endeavors that led me here, almost exactly as was described in the final entry in the mystical ancient book. It was the only way. There was never going to be a roundabout path to get here, a shortcut, a properly placed bridge over the obstacles below, or a way to just find it or discover it easily, to bypass all of the steps required to arrive where no one had ever gone before. And, if there was, then this wouldn't have been the correct path anyway. It would not have been my perfect line, nor would it have carried the weight, the meaning, the significance, or have been so glorious in the end.

Legend holds that the Fountain of Youth is a spring that can restore the youth of anyone who drinks or bathes in its waters. The tales of this fountain have been recounted for thousands of years, including writings by Herodotus in the fifth century and The Romance of Alexander in the third century. Additionally, during the Age of Exploration in the sixteenth century, the indigenous people of the Caribbean spoke of the water in the mythical land of Bimini. And the prominence of the Fountain reached a pinnacle when, during his travels in 1513, Juan Ponce de Leon was told by Native Americans that the Fountain of Youth was in Bimini, and it could indeed restore youth to anyone.

Is there actually a Fountain of Youth? Does it really exist? If so, where is it? And could I find it?

What if there was some truth to these myths? What if the ability to defy time and its effects was not just a theory? What if you had the ability to age six months each year, or to actually gain back or reverse time?

What if you could maintain your wisdom and life experiences *and* your physical and mental youthfulness?

I have always heard that youth is wasted on the young . . . but as I've said before, I'm not so sure that is true.

Perhaps the young simply allow the years to be wasted on them while in pursuit of eventual wisdom, easily gained or not.

For sure, humans are super complex organisms. We are literally made up of trillions (with a 'T') of cells, each with very specific structures and functions. Some scientific estimates put the number at thirty trillion or more, in fact. That's a difficult number to comprehend and even more difficult to count! Even more miraculous is how grandly these mass universes of cells are orchestrated in perfect harmony for each human body to carry out its basic functions of life.

On top of that, there are believed to be even more bacterial cells than human cells, along with nearly 200 other types of cells. The body is host to nerve cells or neurons, skin cells, fat cells, erythrocytes or red blood cells, brain cells, and so many others. And these cells are each highly specific in their nature and function.

Accordingly, it's vital to point out some of their human functions that are quite unique. For instance, the cells in the repository system are tasked with receiving oxygen and distributing it as carbon dioxide. The physical nature of each type of cell is intriguing as well. Take the brain cells, which are longer in order to effectively transmit brain signals more effectively and efficiently, and the heart cells, which need significantly more energy and get an extra supply of mitochondria to support that need.

Finally, all of these intricate cells work in unison, like an orchestra rising in the perfect pitch, providing uniformity to allow the human body to function effectively. It's simply remarkable when you really think about it. Additionally, it is estimated that all of these cells die and regenerate at a pace that would allow all of them to be replaced completely over a several-year timeframe. If that is the case, then over that period, I would literally become a different person.

Let's say I agree with this assessment. Then that claim makes me ask: What person do I want to be five years from now? I'm not talking just about spiritually, or socially, or the personality in which I wish to elevate. I'm literally talking physiologically—my cellular and physical presence.

Am I going to regenerate my cells with quality replacements as I work to resurrect my body and all of its internal elements each day? Am I going to replenish them with as many as I lose each day?

Is this actually possible, and what makes it so? If it is possible, how do I initiate this cycle effectively and perhaps make it seamless or natural?

I've always thought that we are born, grow up, live our lives, get older, and then eventually die.

I still believe that, of course.

But as it turns out, it's just not that simple.

There are many, many factors that determine the scale, timeline, process, and effect of time, things that design the pattern of the life process—and, ultimately, everyone's path. This is a conversation and conceptualization greater than that of philosophical discussions regarding the choices we make and the wisdom and experience, encounters and relationships we endeavor. This is a pursuit of our physical reality—our actual tangible physical presence of body.

Over time, I began to develop a theory that there just might be some things we do that determine what our cellular resurrection looks like—both internally and externally. It's kind of like the ultimate not-artificial-intelligence-re-creation-ability system.

And, as you can gather by now, it became my life's work to uncover any truth to that possibility. And guess what? There wasn't just one or two things that impacted my cellular resurrection but many, many things. In fact, there is a whole host of factors and characteristics, which in itself is daunting, to say the least.

Again, it's a difficult concept to grasp; however, the grasping, as it turned out, was actually the easy part.

As my research grew and many talented people contributed their expertise to the research, the evidence continued to mount. Not only did the theory have merit, but it began to show itself clearly. It was an extraordinary picture, a brilliant work of art unfolding before me.

There came a point when it actually began to lead me. No longer did I need to stress and tug to pull each little detail out and stress to fit it into my theory. On the contrary, the vision of a glorious masterpiece began to put itself together right in front of me.

I know, I get it. Please stay with me. It really was everywhere. I could actually see it weaving itself together. Like a transparent vision of how all the elements fit together, aligning themselves flawlessly with energy, light, and beauty. The body and mind broken down into bright lights filled with poignant road maps that connected, with even brighter lights for each system of road maps, all strung together like stars in the universe.

But what did all of this mean? I wasn't losing my mind—or, at least, I hoped not.

Was I even meant to see this, and why hadn't I seen it before? For that matter, who else has seen it, and why haven't they shared it with the world?

I have always heard from different sources that we are all connected in some way or another, and I guess I just thought that was a little out there, but now I think differently. I have come to the conclusion that not only are we all connected out there in the world, but we are even more connected *within* ourselves. There is this inner cosmos, majestic and wondrous to see and experience, and even greater to discover. I decided to spend the rest of my days uncovering this mystery, becoming the person I was meant to be as I unlocked these mysteries of the human body.

During my studies, I learned that almost all of this information is everywhere. It's available for all to see and apply in their own journey, ready to fit together like puzzle pieces. However, as I would also come to see, not only is the information elusive at times and tricky to coordinate, but, in many situations, it is in direct competition or conflict with itself. The knowledge has become so convoluted that it has taken a life of its own. At best, it's confusing. At worst, it's at complete odds with itself.

For instance, the medical world is so complicated that it is challenging for one area of study to align itself with another. Science isn't much better as it competes for the answers to so many questions.

Don't get me wrong, I applaud the genius minds in both of those fields and the work they continue to do as they dream to uncover answers and advance humankind. But this is another story. This is the story of how humans arrived in this convoluted information state, why, and what we are to do about it. In fact, I came to the conclusion that as science and medicine accumulate all of the answers, gain ultimate knowledge toward truth that they too one day will arrive back at the very beginning.

Now that I could see this pattern laid out in front of me, this hidden and somewhat slippery vision that was difficult to hold onto, I really liked what I was seeing. But what was I to do with it?

That became my challenge.

I could see this vision, my theory in galvanizing brilliant energy all around me, but I still was not sure how to grasp it and contain it. As it turned out, I would need to learn yet another lesson that made me promise, once it was revealed, I would share it with the world.

The implementation of that promise was overwhelming as I continued my research. The medical and scientific teams assigned to this research effort believe that the science leads to a formula that acts as a prescription, providing the ability to improve everything regarding time and aging and cellular resurrection. Part of the formula seems to be learning or understanding how to count differently, how to calculate this regeneration of physiologies relative to time, and how that, in turn, relates to each of us individually.

For instance, let's look at how we understand time historically. From the time our mother delivers us, we begin the aging process. Every sixty seconds, we age one minute exactly; every sixty minutes, we age one hour exactly; every twenty-four hours, we age one day exactly; every three hundred and sixty-five days, we age one year exactly, and so it goes—year, after year, after year, after year.

Everyone is exactly the same. We each get the same amount of time in a minute, an hour, a day, a year, or a decade. It's the same for everyone . . . or is it?

What we came to extrapolate is that it's actually not the same.

Let me emphasize . . .

In no way do all people receive time the same.

What are some of the factors that affect the pace at which we experience time was the question. In order to find the answer, I started assembling this initial outline in which to base this hypothesis:

Genetics
Nutrition
Activity
Refreshment
Sun
Alcohol
Smoking
Stress
Sleep
Mentality
Balance
Spirituality
and so many others . . .

Wrapping up my thoughts about how we experience time, I realized all of the strength and concentration needed to rappel through the trees was more challenging than I had expected, testing my abilities at each new level as I pushed my feet off the rock, held on with every ounce of energy to the rope sliding through my hands, remaining in control until the next fateful push. Even with my dedicated preparation for this climb down through the trees, the jungle was never going to give in without a fight. So, now that I'm here on the jungle floor, I lean up against a tree to spend a few seconds gathering myself. Although, literally moments away from realizing my dream, I'm feeling a little light-headed, which leads to a near daydreaming state. As I stand there, my thoughts begin to race all over the place and eventually toward all the effort that has gone into this process of understanding the universal structure that contains all the necessary commodities allowing us to grasp the simplicity of human functioning regardless of their attempts to evade.

When I come back to earth and regain control of my surroundings, the light is brighter, more powerful now. That's all there is at this point—just light. My heart is still beating rapidly, but not out of fear anymore like when I first descended through the tunnel of treetops. It's now more from a pure chemical release of endorphins, adrenaline, enhanced blood flow, and oxygen to the brain. I am more alive than I have ever been.

How do I hold onto this moment? Is it even possible?

I begin to open my eyes very, very slowly . . .

The light begins to crest through my barely opened eyelids. It spreads and grows, larger and larger . . . and then, with my eyelids now open about halfway, the outer edges of the light begin to reflect additional colors. They are more vibrant—and they are growing. The center of the light is white, with a pallet of colors growing, greens, blues, yellows, all the colors of the rainbow.

My eyes are fully open now, but I'm not sure what I'm seeing.

Perhaps I'm having trouble seeing after keeping them closed so tightly for such a long period. I rub my eyes and obtain greater control of vision, and the odd shapes of light begin to come into view: a Sage, a philosopher, a physiologist, a counselor, a parent, an advisor, a spiritual guide, a child, a teacher, an intellectual . . . figure after figure comes into focus. I'm overcome with emotion and tears run down my face.

With my eyes fully open, everything else comes into clear view, and it's beautiful. The entire area is pristine, as if untouched, really untouched, seemingly unchanged since the beginning of time. It looks like a garden with trees and flowers adorned claiming vivid colors. I follow a stream that runs through the green field until it ends at a small pool of water.

I close my eyes and open them again to make sure I'm not seeing things.

I'm not seeing things.

The pool is shining back at me! It is reflecting light in thousands of directions like a diamond. It measures between six to nine meters across in a sort of a sphere. The water is completely still, not a ripple of any kind to be seen other than in the precise center of the pool where there is a tiny expression bubbling up from the water, no more than a few centimeters high, seemingly coming from a gentle push underneath the surface.

As I draw closer to the crystal pool, the light begins to reflect off me. It's almost blinding, and I find it very hard to see. But once again, I'm not afraid. I feel highly charged and totally at peace. I look down at my hands and arms and see they are reflecting the light and that light is also bouncing off of the mountain face, the rocks, the trees, and the leaves all around me.

I'm trying hard to make out the image in the reflections that I keep catching glimpses of. I continue to turn and look in different directions, but I see the same reflections rebounding from the rocks and trees above . . . from everywhere.

I look down, and it's the same thing—more of the same reflections.

I still can't make out the image clearly. It's like one of those holograms where you see the picture as it appears overtly at first glance; however, if you look deeper with a highly concentrated focus, you can make out the image underneath, and it's a completely recognizable image of something totally different.

So, I try to focus with that same intensity. To look past the obvious picture that I'm seeing when using my normal sight and see beyond the surface of the reflections.

After several minutes of focusing, the vision deep inside the reflections starts to appear. Everywhere I look, I can see it. It's perfectly clear now. Shaking, I drop to my knees in slow motion and simply sit on the ground.

In near disbelief, I clasp my hands together as if to pray. I feel a tear slide down my cheek. I'm actually here. I really discovered it. For all eternity man has been searching for this place in hopes of changing his and I have arrived.

This discovery changes everything.

The real question is how to encapsulate it and share it with the world.

I approach the pool and gently bubbling fountain for a closer look, and it begins to change. I take another step closer, and then another. The pool starts to crystalize and appears to have hardened to the surface, yet the center bubble remains.

Confused and not sure I believe what my eyes are presenting to my brain, I am drawn closer with a desire to be in the presence of this site. A spirituality is revealed. A reverence is demanded, and accepted, with ease.

Gently reaching down to touch the water, or what I thought to be water, I realize that it is more like a hard surface, a solid pool of crystal. I extend my left index finger having already discarded any belongings, reaching forward to prod the surface of the water with the very tip, not sure what the encounter might bring or what risk it may entail.

Would it burn? Is it sharp? Would it be freezing?

The weather is cool, around sixteen degrees Celsius; however, the pool surface looks very cold, perfectly pure like ice. It is piercingly shiny and bright, highly welcoming, drawing me in. I don't want to resist, but I'm not sure if I would be able to regardless. When my finger finally touches the surface, it feels like glass or a diamond with the same temperature as the surroundings.

And I find myself walking out, on the surface like something from a Bible story. I feel secure, at peace. No words are needed, and I stand there, wondering what comes next. Am I just supposed to stand here? Should I close my eyes, pray, sing, kneel, breathe, yell?

Not knowing what's expected of me, I stand without moving, and there is utter stillness (except for the tiny bubble still gently flowing as if it were the brain center or perhaps the heart)—if there is such a thing. I remain calm and collected, not wanting to even increase my heart rate. A lifelong practice of meditation training kicks in and I just close my eyes, cross my hands with ease, and begin extremely slow breathing exercises to enable calmness.

One of the things I had become accustomed to during my meditation practice was focusing on the present and nothing else. It did not come naturally or easily. It took a very basic conditioning effort and a great deal of consistent practice to gain strength, day after day. I learned to focus completely on my inner thought pattern with only one peaceful picture absolute and total in my mind. Nothing else can enter during this state. It's where I find total and absolute peace—a release and a fullness.

Wait, something is starting to happen . . . I try not to get distracted, to stay in my present with eyes closed, relaxed and breathing slowly and calmly. I feel as if I'm slowly sinking into the pool, but I'm not sure. Anxious to see what is going on around me, I open my eyes. To my amazement, I discover that I haven't been sinking into the pool at all. . . it has been rising up around me, consuming me. I look at my arms, hands, legs, and feet and see that my entire body has been consumed and is now shining. This crystallized vision is everywhere—including my entire body. The garden is no longer visible. Actually, nothing is. Everything everywhere appears to be connected, including a specific connection to me. Somehow I have become one with the crystal pool, or it's consumed me, or something of that nature. It's beautiful and calm and spectacular.

I begin to understand the message now. I close my eyes again and slowly walk backward out of the pool—or off of it, as the case may be.

As I clear the edge of the pool, I open my eyes to take another look at the surroundings, and the vision is gone. No lighted reflections or crystals shining or diamonds. I'm back in the peaceful garden again. I walk to the edge of the garden and lean against a large stone rock to reflect on what just happened.

How long was I in the crystal state? It seemed like it was only seconds, but actually almost six hours had passed!

What was the message? What am I now supposed to understand that I had not before?

Pulling out my diary to log everything that had just happened, finish my notes about the last couple of weeks and, of course, attempt to encapsulate the culmination in the crystal pool would be exhilarating and tiring, but I knew the timing is crucial for the scientific record. However, I'm not sure that I was prepared for the complete onset of emotional release that would ensue. I sat in the garden for several more hours with thoughts coming at such a pace that I could not write them down fast enough. Overcome with revelations, I wasn't even thinking really. Words were simply pouring from my mind onto the page in illuminating detail.

Calmer after finishing my notes, I recognized that this experience had eclipsed all of the previously declared expectations. A grander climax than any I had envisioned.

As I travel back to the institute, my mind is racing, trying to figure out how I will explain this discovery. The evidence is absolute and compelling, but it still takes tremendous faith, beyond basic intellect, to grasp the gravity of these findings. We as a society have become so accustomed to accepting the obvious, the clear space right in front of us that we have a truly hard time understanding the simplest, most basic of realities.

When I return to IHAC to reveal the results of my experience in the garden and the diamond pool, all of my individual travels seem to have merged into one rather than the many different explorations they were. There was a connection from one to another, a bridge, if you will, an acknowledgment that you really couldn't continue without the others to provide take-off and landing points.

Now that the final discovery destination spot is behind me and initial information shared with the research leaders, I head to Switzerland where a newly formed team of medical and scientific experts have assembled to take a deep dive into my exposure to this site. They mean to see if there are identifiable, measurable results from my exposure to this pool—and perhaps find some explanations as well. It will take a lot of convincing for them to get a handle on what I've seen and their investigative processes will be thorough which is exactly what is needed to gain actionable and publishable support within the research, scientific, and medical societies at large.

After several days of debriefing and downloading a year's worth of information for the organized panel of ancient civilization experts, who have also come to Lausanne, and discussing what it all meant, the next steps became obvious to everyone.

Many tests would be run on my body and mind. There would be physical and mental examinations, of course, as well as numerous scans, blood and cell diagnoses, magnetic pulse field tests, and much more. I would be prodded and probed and scanned and imaged and run through an exhaustive examination process. To say there was a magnitude of skepticism was an understatement, but that was actually welcome as ultimately this entire journey was about finding real, identifiable, and reportable results. If all of this work led to just another theory, that would not be the worst outcome; however, it would pale in comparison to discovering verifiable, factual, discernable, actionable, publishable processes that could change the world as we know it.

I was prepared to undergo significant examination and exhaustive tests myself, as I was the only one who experienced the transformational changes, and it was critical to determine the pool's impact. There were numerous tests, physical examinations, extensive notes, physical materials, pictures, drawings, writings, my diaries, maps, imagery, etc.

Without question, this discovery—having taken decades—will be perhaps the greatest ever recorded. Accordingly, we have to get it right. Documenting each and every detail, no matter how small or difficult, is vital to the further evolution of mankind and perhaps its survival.

Actually, the resurrection aspect is a greater declaration of what this means. Accordingly, we have to be even more thorough because if we were to miss something or leave holes in the theories, there would be a resulting loss of time, life, and health—literally. This work is perhaps the most important ever conceived or conducted. It's larger than any one human or group, organization, or even country. We must get it right and call on any and all available knowledge and talent to make sure that we do.

Upon completion of the extensive two month-long process (that was sure to only be the beginning of the inquiries that were to last decades), an initial conclusion was reached, and it in fact changes the landscape of almost everything we've ever known in our present day society—social norms, health treatments, lifestyles, nutrition . . . everything.

Once the publications were complete and approved by the team and societal heads, we moved to have the announcements about the discovery made live from the United Nations Educational, Scientific, and Cultural Organization headquarters in New York City. The years of study to follow would begin the marriage of science, medicine, humanity, spirituality, and the magic of the human spirit in a completely new configuration. Straightforward processes of coordination and communication would be created allowing these platforms to offer cohesive support of the findings. In time we would all come to understand that what happened to me in that special place was a miraculous discovery, perhaps the discovery of all time.

The secrets of the Fountain were not on the island of Bimini, nor in Africa, Mesopotamia, the Ancient Indus Valley, the Mayan Civilization, Greece, or China; yet, they did offer the guide to its discovery. The Fountain of Youth, the actual physical Fountain of Youth, was located inside the complex makeup of the human body and mind. The water, fluids, chemicals, and magical potions needed to continually rehabilitate the human organism exist deep down in the cellular and molecular construction of each and every human. The makeup and configuration of the physical human body and mind is a most astonishing laboratory and is created with all of the special components of the Fountain of Youth and it will continuously reproduce itself when it follows the principles by which it was originally designed. We can complicate, interrupt the process, or restrict its natural procedural intent by not allowing these natural cycles to occur. Or we can simply accept its perfect design and follow the anciently prescribed instructions.

I'm not talking about some fanciful spirit stream of existence. I'm talking about real science and the sui generis, the architectural construction for which we were all created. Our bodies and our minds will live for eternity on this earth and beyond, and they have the talent and ability to resurrect themselves over and over and over again. They can push the reset button when we incorporate the principles, that we have hidden away and over many, many generations, lost the ability to do.

The Fountain of Youth is real. The diamond pool is real. The science is real. The ability to own it is real.

After exhausting every complicated concept from the masters, it seems undeniably simple now.

I need to go back to the beginning.

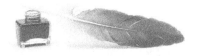

Chapter 7

THE COMPOUND

THE ANCIENT MESOPOTAMIA
CIVILIZATION

H ere I am, back at the beginning—or at least the beginning as best we know it from excavations and subsequent in-depth inquiry and declarations along with countless dissertations presented over hundreds of years.

The result of this journey to Mesopotamia was a trip back in time some twelve millennia to 10,000 BC—the age of the oldest recorded civilization. The Mesopotamians were a historic civilization situated among the Tigris–Euphrates river system in the historic region of Western Asia. The Mesopotamians believed that they were as close to God as humanly possible. That they were truly divine and in the presence of ultimate truth.

To be fair, Mesopotamia is the site of the earliest developments of the Neolithic Revolution. It led to some of the most important developments in human history, for example, the invention of the wheel, the development of cursive script, and agriculture. But the purity and simplicity by which these people lived brings me to the truest of crossroads.

What would it all mean, and how does the way they lived impact lives in the centuries that followed?

Today starts the last leg of my journey. You would think I might be depleted from over a year of this travel extravaganza that has taken me literally all over the world, but that's not the case. In fact, I've gained strength at every turn. Even during the times when I felt like I had lost my way, or felt like I was on a wild goose chase, something kept me going strong.

Sure, there were some days when I was so exhausted I could barely lift my eyelids, but then those times specifically ended up being the best periods of rest as I leaned back against a mountainside or a tree next to a roaring river or lay down in a field staring up into the heavens.

You see, there was nothing and everything all at the same time. That may seem impossible, but purely by chance—and the stubbornness to never give up my quest—I found an evolving strength each and every day. The task list that would normally overwhelm me seemed simpler, more easily processed, yet the accomplishments were greater and grander. Conditioning had become innate for me, instinctual. A natural process, a state of being, a lifestyle. Not a robotic one, mind you. It was quite the opposite; it was a really enjoyable effort to be in the present continually. That's not easy for anyone, I promise, but it was worth it.

By removing all the layers, distractions, interferences, negative mind drain, and disruptive behavior that came from being led to be the way I thought I should be in society, most of my disruptions began to fade away.

Accordingly, during that conditioning process, the layers of strength began to present themselves as if they were bands of muscle, one wrapped over the other, strung together like vines woven magically around each other, growing for many years until they are unmatched in unity and strength. Thicker and stronger the vines grow, yet they remain pliable and youthful, fresh and vibrant to the eye. They become not only fiercely supportive, but perhaps unbreakable. My layers of strength were just the same. My ability to own my task or station became inherently known to me and, in time, to everyone around me. I didn't need to say anything, so I didn't. I just expressed it internally and lived it out in my daily life. However, I think it was obvious to most around me that something was different.

It was a feeling of being reborn, resurrected, and completely confident in the steps I would be taking as I moved forward each day. Amazingly, that feeling also came with a calm and humility of sorts. The need to impress or design my life around another's perspective or opinion was continually dissipating, and instead, there was a desire to be joyful in myself.

It is no understatement to say that it was a long road from there to here, but it was worth it for sure. I felt complete satisfaction in not arriving at my goal, which was no longer a goal anyways. Instead, the goal has become to be *continually arriving*. This whole experience has made it illuminatingly clear that it is the journey alone that is the goal. Of course, that may sound trite; however, it takes on a different meaning when every day is impacted with as great of a significance from being in the journey as the attainment of a goal itself.

In the several months following my transformative experience in the jungle ruins and crystal pool, many things have changed in my life.

My spirit was rejuvenated—more than that, it was enlightened and refreshed. I developed a new energy and outlook on literally everything. My energy alone was that of someone who was numerically decades younger.

But that's not all. It's so much more than that. Something happened to me during the several hours I was consumed by the luster of that mystical place.

I'm not talking about a feeling or an emotional or spiritual awakening. Those for sure took place and were formally recorded in my diary within minutes and continuously through the elaborate examinations of my being, inside and out; however, this was deeper. The changes I'm experiencing are real, physical, and physiological. Serious developments have occurred—and continue to occur.

The first thing I noticed after returning to my consistent daily activities was the change in my vision. I had worn reading glasses for years, but I found I did not need them anymore. I had a pain in my knees that disappeared. My strength had increased significantly. I had always been a runner and fitness enthusiast and over the years had slowed down somewhat, but that was no longer the case. I was running fast again—really fast. Some of my logged times were the best of my life.

My physical form had even changed. I looked like a much younger person in appearance for sure, but it wasn't just my appearance. I didn't quite understand it all, but it was more. I was *becoming* something different. My skin had become more elastic, clearer. My sunspots dissipated.

The changes became so dramatic that I knew I had to gain a deeper understanding of what was happening to me. I reached out to the lead researcher from our Switzerland team to schedule a meeting. Knowing that a summit was being coordinated for all of the teams to convene there, I wanted to get ahead of those meetings near Lake Geneva, so I booked my flight.

During our meeting, I showed him the changes I was experiencing, along with notes, pictures, videos, test results, and specific identifiers of the actual changes that were recorded, including brain wave testing, blood flow analysis, protein levels, immune system responsiveness and strength, white blood cell count and other objective indicators and critical biomarkers. . . all recorded by top specialists in each specific area. All of the experts were able to stay in contact through a collaborative agreement and a sophisticated system of data accumulation and coordination to review their findings in real-time, sharing the information from their continual monitoring of the changes I was experiencing.

The teams had been reviewing all of the data prior to my arrival and previously recommended another summit that included the original researchers and the specialists who were monitoring my progress. All of the scientists were provided a consolidated report of the findings from my mystical pool experience in the garden so they could analyze and express their relative understanding of the ongoing result accumulation prior to this highly anticipated summit.

The conclusion they came to, with a great deal of skepticism and reluctance I might add, was that something did indeed happen to me during that fated experience and it was growing more difficult to deny. My rejuvenating and natural rehabilitative processes had started to accelerate on a constant basis.

It was a little nerve-racking . . . and I wondered what was happening to me.

But it was also so exciting that at the most basic level I had an energy that kept me going at a pace that was exhilarating. My sleep patterns were more consistent, and I was enjoying greater levels of rapid eye movement sleep activity. When I woke up, I was fully rested, excited to get up and pursue my day, vividly remembering my dreams.

Even more fascinating was that my hair was more of a natural color than it had been in years, as well as being fuller. My fingernails grew at a more rapid pace than they had for many years. My teeth were whiter and stronger. My bone structure was measuring at a greater density as the year went on. My muscle tone had improved to a level it hadn't been for decades, returning to what it was when I was at my fittest and participating in a consistent pattern of significant physical activity. Even though I have never had an obesity issue, I also became more naturally thin, finding it almost impossible to gain, what I referred to as bad weight anymore. My diet had become more consistent and manageable.

All the tests showed that my metabolism had accelerated, causing an increase in energy processing with an enhanced food processing cycle. My DNA was registering positive instructional development and enhanced reproduction effects. My agility had improved, along with increased coordination and functional movement allowing me to maneuver in ways I hadn't been able to in many years.

The medical doctors conducting the examination were astonished that all the organ, blood, and other internal tests were recording drastic disparities from my years of medical records. In fact, they were concerned that the testing was mistaken. A great deal of cross-referencing was requested followed by the understandable verification necessary to ascertain that these were my actual records and not that of another person or compromised in some way, and that no errors had been made in the collection and analysis. Of course, as it turned out, they were all confirmed to be accurate and the discussions moved along with greater confidence.

After several months or more of the same types of research, the final declaration by the committee was that I had experienced a deep transformative change while in the presence of what has now been termed the diamond pool that was causing real, identifiable changes—an increased cellular regeneration of my internal and external organs. Many theories began to develop to explain these phenomena, from some sort of chemical reaction, to cosmic gases that may have been present, a spiritual awakening of some type, to a deep state of sleep allowing exposure to a greater part of the brain than humanly common and even a time shift or travel, such as how astronauts are believed to age slower during space missions, hence even invoking the Theory of Relativity and on it went. Most enjoyable to me was seeing all of them and their extreme need to understand and explain with actual words and formulas this 'other world' development. It's probably human nature to be ultra-curious and to have answers to gain comfort in our space which is fine; however, it may sometimes create obstacles on the way to accepting and appreciating life experiences. I was confident that we would get there because I was the one that experienced all of this while these experts are all having to imagine it and gain the knowledge with the tools that have guided them throughout life. A significant disadvantage, in my opinion.

Science and medicine have all types of sophisticated, hard-to-pronounce academic names and definitions for what they believe has happened, even though each of them maintains their belief in silos of research and fundamental understanding of the results. Which was to be expected. That being said, considering the differing educations, backgrounds, and cultural influences, I have never been more impressed with a group of professionals. They wanted to learn what the others knew and willingly shared their knowledge with one another. The excitement was so palpable that you could taste it, and egos were accordingly checked at the door. Of course, it didn't start that way, as everyone tends to have very strong opinions, but as the results became more and more evident, intellectual curiosity took over. And everyone gathered around one goal: to determine, grasp, explain, understand what had transpired during this fateful experience. A human being's brain tends to believe that we can write something down, get our heads around the subject at hand and actually grasp what happened and then develop a plausible explanation. So, not surprisingly, that led to some significant frustration for almost everyone because they were all in the business of explaining really difficult-to-explain characteristics and phenomena. However, this one might have been a little out of the norm compared to their usual studies.

As the conference concludes, I pack up my bag and plan to head back to the hotel for a much-needed rest. As I finish packing, someone knocks on the door. In comes one of the lead researchers, a brilliant Indian scientist from Kolkata I met earlier during a round of the testing procedures. She oversaw and conducted some of the examinations. She softly asks, "Professor, excuse me, do you have a moment?"

I stop my organizing efforts and say, "Of course, how may I help you?"

"Would you be willing to visit with me for a few minutes? I have something you need to see." Although calm, she seems anxious, so I agree.

We go to her lab on the other side of the campus. Her lab is like most, immaculate and clinical with several testing tables and the traditional scientific and medical paraphernalia you might expect.

We sit down at one of the tables to sip on tea that she politely pours. She starts with some small talk, asking about my experience thus far, how my trip was, my thoughts of the city . . . clearly not divulging what is actually on her mind. Seemingly ill at ease for some reason.

After visiting for fifteen or twenty minutes, a fairly uncomfortable pause and total silence overcomes our conversation, as I look around the room, wondering what she wouldn't say. Finally, I break the silence with, "Thank you doctor . . ."

At the same time, she chimes in with, "My analysis uncovered more."

I pause before asking, "More . . . what?"

"My laboratory results concluded something different than what you have been presented with over the past few days. Something else is showing up in my work."

I listen, my attentiveness growing.

She opens one of the folders she had been fumbling with and pulls out a paper about three centimeters thick. Keeping her hand on top of it, she slowly looks at me and says, "This is what I believe happened to you."

Now she has my attention.

Totally engaged at this point, I hang on every word.

She opens the paper and points, "Okay, look at this. This isn't normal, or at least not what I usually see from these categories of tests. Your individual results show that your cells are multiplying."

"What do you mean?" I ask.

"Here, look, you see how this graph turns up and crosses over the timeline right at your date of arrival in the jungle pool area." Her speech pace begins to increase, an excitement in her voice, clearly gaining confidence in her presentation. "And look at these charts as well; they show the same thing. All of them converging at the same point. I've never seen this before. On some very rare occasions, there may be some similarities, but these are all exactly the same. More than thirty different test results conducted by different professionals with different input and varying testing methods from research labs all over the world."

"When I plugged all of the results into the formula and changed only the input of the time construct, every single one of them came back with the exact same results. They intersect at the exact time of your recorded entry into the pool. That's not possible. I ran them over and over again. Come over here and look through this microscope at the cell growth, then look here at this time lapse presentation of the same cells as they are sped up in rapid succession."

"Okay," I said. I'm curious, but I'm obviously still not getting it.

To which she exclaimed, "Professor, these are your brain cells!"

"So . . . what are you saying?" I asked.

"I'm saying that these test results prove that something happened to you during your experience."

I chimed in instantly, "I'm aware that something has been changing and that I've been affected by my journey in measurable ways."

"No, that's not it. Something significant happened to you at this exact moment. Something highly unusual. Something out of this world has transformed you inside and out. You are not the same anymore. You are a different person. I mean, I know that you are the same person, but your physiology is different and it happened at that exact moment, as if you were instantly struck by something or something entered you creating an instantaneous change physically."

She goes on to describe the experience that I had during my visit on the jungle floor as a part of theoretical physics, basically by using various mathematical models and abstract physical objects and systems to explain what is, in actuality, a more natural phenomenon. In other words, what happened to me wasn't unusual at all. It's a natural experience for the human body; however, in my particular case, it happened in just an instant when I was in the jungle.

I need some time to absorb what has just been unveiled and what it all means. Why did it take the interaction with the pool to create these effects, or at least for them to be obvious to me as well as those around me?

Once back at the hotel, I look at some notes from about a year ago at the beginning of this fantastical journey. They were given to me by someone I admired for his dedication to a theory with the goal to control time, to maximize the amount of completeness of your time on this earth. The dreams, enjoyment, fulfillment, relationships, experiences, overall health and fitness, a sort of hyper time guided by a state of existence through hyper wellness.

In order to succeed at this goal, he explained, you must be able to own the layers of development in hyper wellness. And in order to own all of the layers, I had to own the first one. And to own the first layer, I didn't need to understand it.

The understanding would come later.

It actually didn't matter if I read his study and believed that I already understood it. Even if I knew what to do and all of the particulars about what it means, it would only matter that eventually I owned it. And in order to own it, I will have to practice. This consistency would allow the corrections necessary to rechart my path. Or at least that's my understanding of his concepts.

Practice? Like when I was younger and practicing for a competition or event?

Confused yet?

I am certainly confused, but then comes the really good part.

It's very simple, as it turns out—the requirement to work toward a consistency of desired patterns. Now I understand. He did not say it was going to be easy; he said it was simple. However, there is an easy part too.

But first, I wonder what the simple part was.

This is where the proverbial rubber meets the road. You learn, or unlearn, over time common things you have heard your whole life, like "more is better." Or you make those many New Year's resolutions that most often go unfulfilled within a few days or weeks after being established.

Trust me, this is a very positive, powerful, and empowering message, so stay with me as I get to the point—his paper continued!

But first, let's get through the tough part. Let's just dive right in.

You have to do less!

What?

Yes, that's right: LESS!

How in the world do we improve our situation or reach our goals by doing less? If I told my significant other that some science guru told me to do less, how would that go over?

Probably not that well, but I would hope that eventually they would get it too.

See, I don't want to ride that roller coaster anymore, especially when it comes to important life processes, things that really matter, like my health or significance.

I remember a friend telling me that one of their family's favorite places to go was an amusement park in America. The roller coasters, of course, were the children's favorite experience, so they went up and down and around a lot. I mean, a lot! For amusement, pure enjoyment, absolute full belly laughter, and entertainment, not much else can compare. They had some memorable times.

However, when it comes to life and dreams and goals, I want to take out as much of the roller coaster part as possible. I recognize that some of the ups and downs are always going to exist and are, in fact, a necessary part of advancement (the perfecting), but I really do want to make it as smooth of a ride as possible. I'm not talking about risk aversion or fighting with every last ounce of energy toward something worthwhile and pursuing your life mission. (That's a later chapter and one of the greatest blessings in life.) If you have experienced just a little bit of life, you already know about the roller coaster to which I'm referring, and this particular ride can be pretty rough.

A few years ago, I visited an amusement park myself. We rode a special roller coaster. It was an old, yet somewhat famous, ride that has been a part of the park's legacy for decades. The wooden track takes you on the traditional twists and turns and back and forth; however, it is rougher than most. That's probably why so many kids are lined up waiting for long periods of time to enjoy it. It was, without question, the worst ride I've ever been on. It literally knocks you all over the place and rattles your whole body.

All that to say, I've done the rattling approach many times in my life (most other people probably have as well) and believe there are other options that may offer greater success. It's so impressive how hard people will work to get to a better spot, to achieve their dreams, to accomplish what they thought about every day as a child—only to fall short over and over again.

I've heard it's insanity to think that you can produce different results by doing the same things you've always done. That may be true in some cases, but in others, the same thing may be exactly what is needed to actually be successful in developing a foundation for something completely different, moving one directly toward those different results.

Regardless, I believe the most important factor is that I am tuned into the right tone, not rattling along or going up and down on a roller coaster. That my receptors are dialed in properly.

This theory sounded a little complicated to me, but as I would find out, just like everything else in the cascading world, it was just the opposite. It was, in fact, very simple, and the simpler I made it, the sooner the results I was pursuing would come and the more effective I would be at achieving those correct sounds.

What sounds? What were the sounds I was being instructed to hear or to seek out? I am intriguingly compelled by this concept; however, first I need to continue digging deeper on battling the complexities of smoothing out my "life path line".

Where do I get this clear intelligence to not just get on the correct path but the one that will allow me to smooth out the line that I am traversing? It's okay that it will be difficult, offering numerous challenges along the way, some bumps, bruises, and even some breaks, as those peaks and valleys will hopefully provide learning opportunities and the ability to change the dials on my craft and correct course toward the believed desired direction. Which is where I have decided to begin. What is the direction that I'm going? Would I recognize it if I saw it or if I ran directly into it while it was smacking me in the face? So, I have to start right there. At best guess, I go in the direction of where I believe

I want to end up. If I'm going to go on a trip to a specific destination, I can pinpoint that spot and develop a plan to get there. Sounds pretty simple, just draw a line from where I am now to the destination that I have laid out as my end goal at this point in my life, and then put in those one, two, three…steps to get there.

Not so fast. Yes, it's true that if I know the destination point and the starting point, I should be able to map out a direction to that point (of course that's some effort in and of itself, but let's save that for later). However, it is important for me to realize that I may not know where I am. Or exactly where I am based on a great deal of inputs. What? Surely, I know where I am. If it's true, that I really do know where I am at this moment in time, really know, then I am likely ahead of most and most definitely on the right path or at least at the right starting point. Why would this be the case? Well for me to truly know where I am, it will take a level of honest introspection that may be trying to my self-esteem. Honestly, it may even be uncomfortable. If I want to get the purest line for mapping my path, then this process must take place, by breaking down the barriers and removing all of the camouflage, protective armor, and taking off the makeup. How will those truths help determine the starting point? Truth will tend to have its own plan, so the experience will likely prove to be illuminating and enlightening providing ultimate freedom to begin the journey.

Once I've received a clearer determination of my starting point, then I am set free to begin dreaming of the possibilities of the roads ahead and the dreams calling my name. A celebration will likely occur during these revelatory pursuits, as many accomplishments and gifts of life will hopefully find their way to the surface as well, initiating a wall of legacy for which to establish the foundation of pillars to support construction.

No matter the size of your legacy, especially as you begin this journey, it is significant.

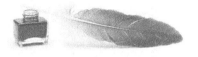

Chapter 8

LIFETONES

BHOPAL, INDIA

Dancing has always been a great joy of mine. From a very young age, the impulse to dance was instinctive. Maybe because it seemed to come naturally to me. I was good at it, so I liked it, or perhaps I liked it so it came more naturally making me work harder at it and become better.

Whatever the case, dancing represented joy and happiness, a certain freedom of expression, and a transition to another place and time. I could let go of the world around me, defy gravity, and take flight.

It's fascinating to hear music, those unique sounds and watch the effects it has on you physically, but it also goes much deeper than that. It also has effects on you emotionally. It is inspiring, energy generating. There is a special release of chemicals inside the brain that can bring us to a different place—a place that lifts our souls and causes us to move, physically move, literally float above our own body.

The art of dance has been recorded as far back as the earliest civilizations, the very birth of humankind. Dance was used in celebratory occasions, rituals, and entertainment. Archeologists have uncovered relics depicting dance that date back to prehistoric times from paintings in India and Egypt, illustrating dancers from the era of circa 3,300 BC, including ethnic and contemporary dances of that ancient period. Dance was used as a social means of integrating with others, and it also may have been used as a survival technique for learning cooperation.

An especially interesting fact about dancing is that more recent studies have shown that talented dancers today share two genes with those who are endowed with social communication skills. I find it fascinating that this passionate expression—natural, pure, emotional, instinctual, and uninhibited—would come from this scientific, anatomical dialogue between the mind, body, and soul.

Even more amazing is the mental response to this feel-good activity. The real energy generated by this anomaly is transferred to the body in a useful form. The effects last for a period of time; however, they last for different periods of time depending on the person. Additionally, the continuation of the process that generated the energy in the first place is required in order to form a conditioning foundation that maintains the energy flow ownership. The continual conditioning of the energy then forces an increase in the effects of the energy on so many parts of the body and mind. It actually grows over time, recruiting and actually encouraging, the enhancement of these positive benefits.

One of the most remarkable sites that identifies the historic declarations of dance is the Bhimbetka rock shelters in Madhya Pradesh, India that descend from the prehistoric Paleolithic and Mesolithic eras. The site shows examples of the earliest life on the Indian subcontinent, during the Acheulian era of the Stone Age. It is located some forty-five kilometers southeast of Bhopal in the state of Madhya of the Raisen District of India. The seven hills and more than 750 rock shelters are cast over an area of ten kilometers, some of which are believed to have existed over 100,000 years ago. These illustrations have been described as a rare glimpse into human settlement and our cultural evolution from hunter-gatherers to agriculture, as well as visual expressions of prehistoric spirituality.

Thinking about these ancient expressions of dance makes me wonder what I'm listening to that impacts my movement, my expressions, my direction. Am I catching the vibe? We are surrounded by sounds. How do these sounds affect my decision-making process? How do they make us move? Is it positive? Do these sounds lift our spirits and make life worth living? Or do we allow sounds to come into our lives that are not positive? Sounds that bring us down and cause us to lose sight of what is most important? Are there sounds of distractions, causing us to lose our way in the night?

Regardless, I believe the most important factor is that I am tuned into the right tone. That my receptors are dialed in properly.

It's a fragile dance that has been with us since the beginning of time. Yet, sometimes, it's violent. I'm continually trying to understand how I can drown out the noise that keeps me from following my path, the noise that controls me, brings negativity and distractions that are clearly a waste of time, and, more critically, might lead me on a path I might not return from.

Now that's a daunting and scary thought.

Through the process of experiencing the cascade and, ultimately, the Fountain of Youth, I had stepped back and reflected on the purity of it all. The utter beauty of pursuing a life filled with purpose, a direction that is different for everyone but filled with a beauty that will please the heart and soul once discovered.

One of the most glorious experiences of life is that all humans are so very different. Yet, there are some common threads, such as passion, desire, love, joy, and excitement that are commonalities in our psychological existence, the will of the mind and soul.

Most of these common threads are present in the lifetones (which became the source and descriptive title of one of my supportive scholarly works that was published from the effect of the Indian exposure), the sounds we hear throughout our lives. These are the actual influences in our everyday life that directly impact the choices we make on a daily basis. They are so powerful (although sometimes silent to the human ear), constantly directing and guiding each and every one of our moves. What I hear, read, receive, visualize, and express determines what I think and how I act and, ultimately, what I will come to believe.

If that is the case, then controlling the sounds and influences around me is the essence of controlling who I will become—or, more precisely, who I am.

The "Lifetone Theories" have concluded that the strong, yet fragile, nature of the human spirit will be guided by the auditory impressions that we decide to play for it. This is not an exaggeration. As beautiful and capable as human nature is, it is so easily influenced. I want to control the input, and the only way to control the input is by identifying where the input is coming from. I want to regularly let in the sounds that guide my life to the right path and draw me in the direction of my dreams, and I want to turn away from those that distance me from them.

When I was developing these experiments, I wanted to conduct them as I would any other of my studies. Accordingly, I needed to define the problem and conduct the initial research on a broad basis with outside input on a broad scale, then narrow that topic to a very specific research question about the desired topic.

First, I start with a hypothesis: Does a specific sound input received directly affect the output of human response and over time design the nature of the subject?

Then I design the experiment, which entails a thirty-day period for listening to sounds, in different physical spaces and settings as identified, conducted at varying times of the day and recording them in a diary with specific detail.

Now on to the data collection stage. This process includes the conduction of the experiment as outlined by the scientist, which includes the collection and recording of the data with extensive notes of the test subject, observations within the natural environment and described settings.

The next step is the analysis of the data. This is the scientific research process of calculating the data with the statistical calculations helping to identify the data and determining if a significant result was found.

And now we move to draw the conclusions. After the data is analyzed, the scientist examines the information and makes conclusions from these findings. The results are compared and contrasted to the original hypothesis and other similarly related experiments, ultimately drawing the resulting final conclusions to be published.

The test subject was me and the period would be one month. I start with a ten-minute session each day with a goal of being still and listening to everything I can. As I begin, I hear a bird chirp, then a leaf rustle, the wind or water trickling. Once completed, notes and reflections are entered into a journal. Each day more of the same, attempting to relax more and listening clearer, searching for new sounds. Over time, I succinctly feel my breathing and learn to clearly hear my own heartbeat. The bird returns each and every day. With eyes closed, it's still perfectly recognizable by the gentle sounds it makes. The bird has found a home, a presence that offers me safety and comfort. Hence an inspiring ritual is born. It is a refreshing light.

As the study continues, I become more aware of the sounds throughout my day, both encouraging and the ones that leave much to be desired. As the theory develops, it becomes very clear how impactful these influences are in my life. The plan is obvious and intentional—to gain the sounds and surroundings that lift my spirit and fill my heart with joy. These results may sound obvious; however, as it turns out, they are not easy to implement in a successful and maintainable way. Accordingly, the philosophies and techniques I learned on my journey would uniquely apply here as well.

For as long as I can remember, I have been aware of this inner process. It has always been there, but I didn't necessarily know how to listen to it or interpret what I thought I was hearing. Honestly, most of the time I just ignored it and thought that maybe I would go there someday when I had enough time to reflect. Kind of like learning a new language or how to paint, or meditating, or actually taking the time to read that book.

Then again, sometimes it was purposeful avoidance behavior or believing that it really didn't matter anyway. I thought it was just my nosy mind interfering with the really important stuff, like all the things that I needed to get done that day, or my very important schedule of to-do lists and tasks. You know, all of those ambitious life plans that would help me get to the top of the ladder, be the best, have prestige and accomplishment, and say 'I made it' according to everyone else's standards.

Later, of course, I understood—to some degree, at least—that what I thought was really important was actually just a load of distractions, things that really didn't mean a whole lot in the grand theme of the play.

Now, after spending more than a year on this special journey, I seem to have made a new friend with my inner self. A really important new friend who isn't a distraction or an interference in my life but *is* forever interwoven in my life. A friend who wants me to do amazingly well and encourages me at every turn.

In fact, this relationship has become symbiotic in nature (although my friend is doing a lot of the heavy lifting by removing obstacles, opening up the doors to positive, uplifting thoughts and feelings, encouraging success, laying out a plan toward a victorious outcome, reducing the clutter). I find so many negative elements routinely being swept aside by the successful relationship I've recently gained. This mental, emotional, and spiritual immune system has taken on a life of its own and continues to get smarter and stronger with each passing day. It is always on guard. Ready to battle. To fight on my behalf.

No, this is not an illusion. It is very real.

My inner self stands as a knight over the land, surveying the kingdom of my life to make sure that I'm protected. Sometimes, of course, I do have to leave the secluded walls of the castle and take on the dreaded monsters that lurk in the shadows. However, I'm never alone in the battle and, more importantly, I'm always prepared.

And I am continually preparing.

Training has become a lifestyle, a daily enjoyment. In fact, it is often the most exciting part of my day. I look forward to the preparation that goes into getting better, stronger, faster. Improving my skills to more successfully pursue my dreams. To be effective and prosper in this pursuit, I must practice.

So, practice I do, and as I practice, I get really good at a lot of very important elements that continue to impact my love of life. I learn that there isn't an ultimate station I want to reach; I just want to enjoy the reaching itself.

Why does it have to be so difficult to reach this status in one's life? To find this place of calm and understanding from within?

I've never really known until this moment.

Just now, it has become illuminatingly clear that this new friend of mine, once upon a time, was actually my enemy. That's right, an enemy from within, a Trojan horse, taking advantage of its freedom and security from inside. Always tricking me.

How did this happen? Why did this happen? Why would I ever let something I assumed I was supposed to control, or that should be naturally accommodating, take advantage in that way?

I realize that it was a trust in the familiar, which began at birth and continued as I grew.

Some might believe that it is a choice; however, I'm extremely confident that it is not a choice. I don't believe for a moment that most people would choose to harbor themselves in negative or oppositional thought patterns, only to fight them off one by one, day after day. I know I try not to allow that space in my head to take over and lead me. I'm strong, and I want to be in control. To be the leader of my own direction and my thoughts, inside and outside of my mind and body. By experiencing the cascade, I finally understood that I wasn't in control all this time—but I could be.

You see, it is not a choice; however, it is a process to be mastered.

I tried this new process. I decided I was only going to allow positive, non-intrusive thoughts, emotions, and feelings to come into my person.

So, I tried. And tried. And tried some more. Unless I was totally engaged in something that consumed me completely, like a completely physically exhausting activity or reading a book that was all-consuming, I had a difficult time lasting one full minute without running off the rails and having to chastise myself with constant reminders, to stop it and think about a beautiful experience in my life. Even then, it was only a matter of moments until I was back in the clutches of this overwhelmingly negative, controlling source. Of course, those were the sounds—the lifetones—deposited into me through all of the environments in my life sphere.

Knowing that it is not a choice, I mean really knowing, is not that easy. It actually was concerning at first, but, later, became comforting. I finally understood, only after experiencing layered cascading, that it is not designed to be a choice, but is, in fact, designed to be a process. And with that came the simplicity of conditioning the process. This meant accepting that I'm supposed to take this very simple path with faith and trust and move forward with the smallest steps possible. The smaller, the better, as they would form the foundation of my strength. It sounds simple, but that is also the challenge.

It's not new to say, that you want to build a house on a rock foundation instead of sand, for it will stand the test of time.

That sounds wonderful although a little trite, but what does it even mean?

I've found that it is difficult to be strong enough, patient enough, or consistent enough to truly maintain a level of simplicity that evolves over time into tremendous power and strength in every facet of my life. I kept making commitments to set goals toward specific desired achievements and put them into motion. With an expressive confidence, I would forge ahead and give it everything I had from the depth of my bones, with the fullness of breath in my lungs and all the desires of my heart set to achieve this next platform, only to find it fading away over time.

It was never a lack of desire or passion or will or energy or love or ambition or caring. Those are all amazing places to be, but they are also very elusive if you think you can just say one of those things and make it so, for it is too grand a thing to accomplish or hold on to for a lifetime.

I learned—and am learning still—that if I could apply a process that was simple, even simpler than the one I just achieved, and the next even simpler, that I would eventually own it and that, ultimately, I could apply that conditioning process to every element of my life and relationships, that I could own them as well. By owning, I mean to truly be in control.

What does this mean in the grand scheme of life? Was I trying to get my head around the thought that I might be able to put a leash on the monster, the enemy inside and repurpose it for my benefit? Could I actually reverse the mental allocation to 85 percent positive and, if so, what would be the result?

I'm not talking about a Pollyanna state of being, for that is not real and that type of expectational thinking may cause you to miss out on the beauty of much of the human experience that we all desire to live. What I am referring to is a state of fulfillment in life and a place of joy that comes from being ever-present and living in the moment. Not regretting the past, or fretting over mistakes I've made, or wishing I could have done better, or worrying about the future and my task list of daily acts. To be here, right now, and know that I am alive and right where I should be at this very moment. Doing what I love, pursuing the dreams that I have right now—and actually enjoying them in the middle of the pursuit.

Of course, everyone's direction is very different, with a unique line that only they can see with purity—eventually. This glorious line is full of fascinating expressions and experiences that strain even the greatest imagination. What type of experience each person has is not key, only that they find their ideal line—their true line.

Since I now know that the conditioning process, the very simple daily focus of exercising, is the key to unlocking the cascade experience, I need to learn where to start. Accordingly, I have to examine what I'm listening to on a daily basis that affects my mentality and my decision-making process.

Many of the roads I traveled were difficult, trying at every turn, urging me to give up. The mountains were steep, the weather unforgiving, the rivers overwhelming, the days long and the nights dark, but I never gave in as relentless as they could be. Why couldn't I accept that everything was pretty good? That I didn't need to challenge all of the gifts I had received? Looking around at so many who had greater challenges than I did, why couldn't I just be thankful for my accomplishments and station in life?

Eventually, it became clear that it wasn't about comparing my life to someone else's at all, but it was about discovering the truest path for me. The ultimate person I could be, getting to know and love that person intimately. There are many parts of a life and a lifetime, no matter the timeframe, but reaching a level of true peace, becoming one with the person I was meant to be in complete fulfillment of my eternal life, is a way of life, not purely a someday hope, but here and now.

This may sound like a state of nirvana, a perfect life. I would say that is true.

It's not the picture of perfection that we tend to assume in the secular world, but it's something real.

Perfection is not everything firing on all cylinders, or looking a certain way, having it all, or any of the other common measurements we see in our day-to-day world. Perfection lies in discovering and living in a place of passionate pursuit, of hope, of faith in a dream so vivid that it releases a chemical high in your mind, body, spirit, and soul. We climb higher, laugh fuller, love greater, sing sweeter, dance freer, learn clearer, sleep deeper, and thrive longer in the journey when we live in that place.

If this sounds unrealistic to you, that's okay. There's more. We also fall harder, struggle often, cry louder, feel deeper, and bleed redder.

That doesn't sound like nirvana at all, does it? But there's the rub: You must know all of the spaces in life and embrace them, love them from a place of total acceptance. We have to go through the full range of experiences to be the greatest versions of ourselves. We experience everything so deeply that it provides a hidden joy we otherwise would have missed. It's similar to a mother's birth pangs, the beauty of delivering one of life's greatest joys from the same place that is causing unrelenting stress and pain.

I like to refer to these experiences as the 'sounds of our life.'

They say that youth is wasted on the young, but I'm not sure that's accurate. I'm just not buying it. The theory my colleagues and I have phrased more clearly is that youth is wasted by the misapplication of time.

For example, I've been working really hard for a long time to improve my health and fitness level. I used to be in great shape. I was very athletic, in fact, but I allowed life to happen. I've never really been much of a follower, continually questioning the norm. Stuff like doing the same things over and over for forty or fifty years and then all of the sudden just stopping was crazy to me. In fact, the word 'retire' in particular is a difficult assertion for me to grasp. Retire from what exactly?

Wouldn't there always be something worth doing, creating, pursuing, dreaming of, or being? I'm a big believer in the concepts of hard work, dedication, and loyalty; however, I just don't think that we were meant to be sheep. It's not healthy, happy, or dedicated to a true balance. It's a sort of imbalance over an entire lifespan.

I've found myself wallowing in ignorant superstitions at times, sometimes for a long time. I would receive input that is off base just a little, primarily from people who are on their own path and are likely, although maybe at a different stage, working to figure it out as well.

Why would I allow that input unless I was completely confident that it is, in fact, allowing me to traverse my correct and true path? Hence the famous Bible verse "As iron sharpens iron, so one man sharpens another" (Proverbs 27:17 NIV) and the importance of identifying the quality of the iron before I use it as a sharpening tool. How many times had I learned of a highly respected line of thought, reasoning, or belief that after a period of time, sometimes decades or even centuries, wasn't accurate at all and a newly adopted concept takes the limelight and becomes the accepted belief for the next period of time?

I needed to learn how to be in control of my best line, my path, which I would do by being in charge of my thoughts.

And to control those thoughts, I needed to control the input of the electrical signals that design those thoughts.

These efforts to control my thoughts, which may include meditation, prayer, breathing exercises, quietness, or relaxation, have been shown to increase cognitive focus and abilities, increase mental strength and self-control, cause a desire for healthy behaviors, remove many of the daily life distractions, solidify relationships, and enhance experiences.

And this proactive concept of being in control of the machine that guides our every movement helps you identify your true line, your individual path.

One highly respected source says not to be anxious about anything but let your requests be made known to God with prayer.

I like to put it this way: Don't worry about anything; just do one thing.

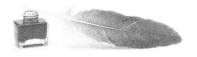

Chapter 9

BREATHLESS

VICTORIA FALLS, AFRICA

Standing up here is truly breathtaking. It took a great deal of effort and was not easy to get here. I had to call in some favors in order to get access to this particular site, but it was worth it. Someone told me one time that they had not arrived, and I certainly have not arrived; however, I like to think that I'm in the process of arriving. Actually, the ultimate arrival, as it were, would be to reach a state of continually arriving.

For what else is there in life that is better than being in a place of completeness at some point during this ultimate journey? And hopefully reaching some important milestones along the way?

Getting as close to the precipice as possible to look over the edge of this massive waterfall is a wonderment.

I can't hear anything as the powerful rush of water consumes and dominates all sounds and in its magnificent glory reaches out and thunderously engulfs everything in its path. It's so beautiful that it takes your breath and your soul away when staring into the abyss.

What a journey, what a climb and a story to tell, but oh so much more to have lived it, so I think I will continue doing just that: living it.

Walking up to the very brink of the roaring water, I can see all the way to the other side of the falls. It's one of the most beautiful sites in the world. I'm not alone anymore, as there are people everywhere to take in the glorious beauty they have heard about, read about, and are excited to see with their own eyes.

It's called 'The Smoke that Thunders,' and it lies on the border of Zimbabwe and Zambia, Tonga: Victoria Falls, Shunga Namutitima, the 'Boiling Water,' the breathtaking massive waterfall on the Zambezi River in southern Africa. It's over 1,700 meters wide and is considered one of the largest waterfalls in the world. Interestingly, it is not considered one of the largest because of a single measurement, as in the tallest or widest, but because of its total size. It's really a fascinating metaphor for my ultimate discovery, which is how to be a complete person, a whole person, the most balanced person I can be.

During the rainy season in southern Africa, the rush of the water flowing into Victoria Falls generates smoke towers that lift hundreds of meters above the crest of the waterfall's edges—a sight that leaves me breathless.

Even more remarkable is how Victoria Falls was created. At the earliest geology, estimated at 150 million years ago, the cliffs of Batoka Gorge consisted of basalt rock. Over time, the melting hot lava began to cool and harden, crack, and eventually created the faults that make up the formation, later receiving deposits from the Karoo and Kalahari river systems, outlining and preserving this rare beauty. Geologists believe that over time, movement in the geological landscape of the central region of

Botswana, which had been flowing south to the Limpopo River, shifted due to a blockage of the Zambezi. Eventually, the lake it was flowing into began to spill over the edges and into the Matesi River and began removing the basalt by breaking it loose one block at a time, leaving the resultant rough edges of the waterfalls unlike those of most other falls.

Amazingly, over the years, the site of the waterfalls has moved eight different times as the river works its way back upstream, from fault line to fault line. They are actually moving all the time, just very, very slowly. So slowly that the movement is not discernible by the eye over smaller periods of time, of course.

I decide to enter the water right before the edge of the waterfall, which is aptly called the Devil's Pool, where many before me have potentially risked going over the edge in embracing the pool. (Although if it's attentively approached with respect and caution, that likelihood is not overwhelming.) Honestly, this is the happiest—no, that's not right—it's the most *joy-filled* moment of my entire lifetime.

Finally, after so many years of searching and believing that my life was meant to be something more, that it was possible to achieve something amazing, I've discovered what I believe to be the most wonderful treasure you could ever imagine. A gift available to all, free, but certainly not automatic. It's special. You have to really want it.

Understand that I didn't say it was hard to obtain, only that it wasn't automatic. You *will* have to pursue it. But if you do, it will come to you with open arms and give you all that there is to offer in this grand scheme of life. I implore you to do just that. Embrace it and accept it as it most definitely is: a gift.

There are many names that could express what this might mean to someone, but none of them are really very important. It only matters that whatever name you give your process inspires you, that your heart is full of joy and complete with passion, and that you desire to achieve all that you were meant to during the years you are awake.

No one really knows how many there are, but there is a finite number for everyone, and you are not just implored but required to jump into that glorious space and own each and every second you are in this place. Right here. Right now. For you should not wait until it is so late. It's never too late while you are here, mind you, but you won't be here forever.

So make haste. Don't just hang on to your dreams. Reach out and grasp them with a relentless grip that will take every ounce of strength you have in you. Drain the blood from your veins if necessary, but grip nonetheless, no matter the cost.

I'm not talking about glory and fame or gold and jewels but loving what—and who—you need to love. What you are called to love.

What you are called to love may include many expressions. In fact, it includes everything except the distractions (which you must respect) that will fall on the road in front of you as you pursue those joys. Don't get me wrong, the fruits of the earth will come, and they may be wonderful accessories to be enjoyed. They are just fun, and that's okay. Part of life and the pursuit is to find the balance of it all, for the stress of controlling every moment is likely worse on your body and soul than the item one is stressing over wanting to control, eliminate, or define.

Here's what I've found to be the best part. The good stuff. It's actually very, very simple to have it all. Although it is critical to define the 'all.'

Once again, it is not easy. But it is so very simple. Perhaps the simplest thing you will ever do.

In fact, the sooner one achieves simplicity the simpler and greater one's life will become. That's why I had to travel this great distance and go back so far. I actually had to go back to the very beginning of civilization, as far as I could, to understand the purity of life. And that culminated with grasping the most basic life and social experiences, how we as a community began to form and learn and grow and share our lives with one another.

I have found a life full of passion and hope, gratitude and expression of faith and fulfillment. I get very emotional these days because of how thankful I am to be here—and to know why.

That's everything: to be here and to know why. It's not so important to know how or even for how long.

The Greeks described it most beautifully. The history of the Greek civilization is dramatic and vast and, of course, full of tragedy and triumph. A historically learned society gave birth to Classical Greece and is considered the birthplace of Western civilization. To the Greeks, science and religion were both entertained in order to get closer to the truth, which meant getting closer to the gods.

However, the most important lessons they taught were about love. In the Greek language, there wasn't just one word meaning love but several. Agapeo or Agape meant unconditional love, as in the love of God in the renewed mind in manifestation. Agape love is also present in a very close family. Phileo was the love between friends. Eros, the sense of being in love, referred to romantic love, and Storge was the love of family, as in a parent for their child or a brother for his sister.

What does all of this mean for my life? Is this the answer to everything?

I believe it may be a grand part of it.

What we spend most of our days doing—where we go and what we pursue—becomes what we love, even if we don't like it. It is our greatest influence on a continuous basis, the greatest number of minutes and hours spent by us, so, of course, over time, it will influence our thought conditioning.

You might say you don't do something because you love it, you do it because it is necessary and the only option you have right now. That is likely true and understandable; however, you must make an effort to cascade beyond that state and reach a new plateau, one where you should be, where you want to be, and where you ultimately belong.

Why do we live, age, and die? Were we meant to live forever? Were we meant to never age or even never die? Who wants to live forever anyway?

If I'm completely honest, I do.

I asked my dear friend how long she wanted to live, and she told me she wanted to live as long as she could impact those around her—the ones she loves and who love her and the ones she is destined to love.

That's quite an insightful wish. I have come to believe that although there are many applications of life and ways in which to spend time, for almost everyone, it is not the time we spend doing all of those things but the people in our lives with whom we spend this time that matters most.

For what is life but paradise? It is everything.

Someone recently asked me: Do you really want to be passionate all the time?

I thought that might be exhausting. Initially, I may have immediately said yes; however, I decided to take some time to reflect and think about the question, and that's exactly what I did.

A number of months spent reflecting and examining this question only provided more questions to contemplate, and, ultimately, that led to a confident response.

First, I began asking myself questions from a contra perspective: What would I not be passionate about in my life? What are the areas of life that I would be okay with just coasting? What about my family? Would I consider not being passionate about my immediate family? Would I consider not being passionate about my health? What about my closest friends or the community in which I live? Would I decide to not be passionate about my faith? Would I choose to not be passionate about my profession or career pursuits or the enjoyment that comes from relaxation and respite? What about the dreams and experiences yet to explore? Or the traveled roads and places I have not gone? Would those plans be considered not worthy of holding onto?

After contemplating a great number of questions in this manner, the answer became very clear. It was a resounding yes: I wanted to be passionate about all areas of my life.

Then I took it a step further to gain a greater perspective of what living a passionate life truly meant. If passion is a strong liking or desire for or devotion to some activity, object, or concept, that would mean that you live in present thought regarding whatever moment you're in. Whatever the activity or lack of activity, I need to be present for it to occur. If I am always present, then I am always living in the current moment, not thinking about the past or worrying about the future. Since the goal is to live life to the fullest, the ultimate goal would be to be ever-present; therefore, living life with passion in all areas would result in ever-present living—or what I have come to appreciate fully as a joyful life!

But we are not talking about a fantasy here. Daily activities are still real, and great effort is needed in our pursuits. When times are hard or things are not going the way we want them to, that passion does not go away. In fact, the harder times should enhance that passion as we are driven by many forces: love, anger, fear, desire, hate, and so many more.

I love my life. I love my solo time, running trails, and thinking and dreaming and breathing deep emotions. I love it so much that it sometimes leads to tears of enjoyment. The physical experience develops a direct link to naturally produced chemicals within my body and mind that are needed, wanted, and sustainable. It's getting high on life.

And it is wonderful. However, nothing comes close to the depth of the love shared with the dearest people with whom I get to share these experiences.

So, what was our life meant to be?

I can only speak for me, but I suspect it's fairly similar for many, if not most.

To express each day with passion toward
our experiences, whatever they may be.

And the 'may be' does, in fact, matter. Sometimes it's not altogether clear during different stages of our lives, but if we simply continue to trust in God and take another step, all of us will find that elusive purpose.

When we ask ourselves what really makes us happy, we tend to think about circumstances, possessions, or the people in our lives. In reality, happiness is an experience that is largely derived from chemicals being released in the brain. Four main neurochemicals, hormones, and neurotransmitters generated in the brain are fundamentally responsible for creating the sensations and emotions that we have learned to associate with happiness.

This is actually great news! It means that even when circumstances, possessions, or people aren't exactly as we'd like them to be, there are simple ways we can increase our happy brain chemicals and alter or elevate our moods.

This is a concept so simple that even mindfulness students in elementary school can really understand it. Parents will tell how their children got a rush (dopamine) from getting an A on a spelling test, or the stimulation (oxytocin) they felt from giving their mom a hug. As it turns out, these chemicals are not just feel-good figments of imagination but real, scientific effects on the human body and mind.

One of the more well-known chemicals our brain produces are endorphins, an opioid neuropeptide, which means it is produced by the central nervous system to help us deal with physical pain. Endorphins also make us feel lightheaded and even giddy at times. One of the ways to induce endorphins is physical movement, such as exercise. In one study, as little as thirty minutes of walking on a treadmill for ten days in a row was sufficient to produce a significant reduction in depression among clinically depressed subjects.

Another of the well-known chemicals is serotonin, and this may be the best-known happiness chemical because it's the one that antidepressant medication primarily addresses. Serotonin is a neurotransmitter that is naturally triggered by several things we can do each day, such as exposure to bright light, especially sunshine, exercise, and happy thoughts. Some research has found that a higher intake of certain foods may bring on the effect as well.

Yet another of these chemicals is dopamine, a neurotransmitter often referred to as the chemical of reward. When you score a goal, hit a target, or accomplish a task, you receive a pleasurable hit of dopamine in your brain that tells you you've done a good job. But you can also get a natural dose of dopamine when you perform acts of kindness toward others. Volunteering has been shown to increase dopamine as well. And some research has even found that it only takes thoughts of loving-kindness to bring on the dopamine high.

And, of course, there is oxytocin, the hormone produced in abundance during pregnancy and breastfeeding. Oxytocin is primarily associated with loving touch and close relationships and is normally produced in one part of the brain and released by another. This hormone provides a multiple whammy of warm fuzzies by stimulating dopamine and serotonin while reducing anxiety. To get your hit of oxytocin drug-free, you can snuggle with someone you love. Man's best friend will even do the trick.

So, if you're like me, happiness may at times feel like the unachievable holy grail of emotion. But luckily, our brains and bodies are constantly undergoing complex chemical processes that we can affect with our daily actions. Once we understand how our feel-good hormones and neurotransmitters work, we may be able to trigger them more easily than we realized.

*"You cannot teach a man anything, you
can only help him find it within himself."*
—**Galileo**

I am learning to do just that. That starts with understanding that beauty is more wonderful than perfection. I came into this world with a heart and a soul and forever that will be.

As I stand on the edge of Devil's Pool, looking out over the gorge, watching the thunderous plummeting of the water hundreds of meters below and the billowing smoke clouds it generates above, my breath is swept away by the overwhelming beauty in every direction. The temperature is perfect, the air is crisp . . . and I'm at peace.

One question keeps popping up in my mind with a demand for answers.

(No, you may not think about it and get back to me. I need an answer now.)

What leaves you breathless?

The question rings out again and again, and I look back on all of my experiences with great wonder. Was it the dreams, the desire of achievement, the dedication and effort put toward victory in an endeavor? Was it the one special person who changed my life forever? Was it the birth of a child? Could it be the continual pursuit of a dream? Was it the loss of a loved one that impacted my world? Was it majestic faith in something greater? Was it the recognition of a life at its last days? Could it have been this journey to find an answer that has been driving me forward for decades? Is it the answer to the truly timeless question of why I'm here and what I was meant to be and who was I meant to touch?

Are those the things that take my breath away?

Standing at the completion of my journey—or perhaps the beginning—I take a deep, purposeful breath, as full as I ever have. It comes in, and I hold onto it as long as I can.

Just before releasing it from my lungs, my breath stops for an instant. For that moment, I'm actually without air. When it goes back out, just prior to the next inhale, it stops again for that same brief moment. I do this several times, breathing in through my nose and out through my mouth, leaving no air in my belly, one more time and then again, and again, feeling absolutely alive and exuberant.

That's when I realize . . . after so many travels, worlds visited, truths discovered and told, falling down, and getting back up again, over and over, cascading to my full potential, I finally understand.

And I am breathless.

THANK YOU

Thank you dear readers for reading to the end of this little tale!

To learn more about the passion journey, how to apply the life principles and conditioning of the "Cascade" and discover the "Fountain of Youth" in your life, please visit us at: timelessthebook.com

ACKNOWLEDGMENTS

It is with the utmost honor and privilege that we would like to thank Morgan James Publishing and its leader David Hancock, along with the amazing support team at MJP, who have led us down this path with encouragement and expertise at every turn. We are grateful for the opportunity and the journey afforded us. To Aubrey Kosa, our editor, who is wise beyond her years and patiently shares her talents of the "Tangling Words" with total passion and a caring heart.

We would also like to share our appreciation for the artistic abilities of several individuals: Rachel Lopez for the beautiful and meaningful TIMELESS cover design, Elli Tennant for sketching the traveler's vision in the "Four Pillars" image, and Bess Garison for lending her creative eye to the authors photograph.

To each other, it has been the blessing of a lifetime to have met you, knowing that a journey as blessed and wonderful as ours could only be achieved with true love and dedication.

About the Authors

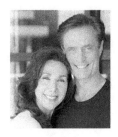

Kathy Brook has created a highly accomplished and inspirational 20-year career as an elite health and wellness trainer and coach. Her philosophy has always been that she never sees age, just the heart and soul of her clients. As a former professional runway model, Kathy continues to pursue her love for fashion, lifestyle, and nutrition as she expands her KathyBrookWellness brand.

Victor Brook is an entrepreneur and investment manager, with a background in business development. As a former stockbroker, college football player and model, he has continued to nurture his expertise and passion for athletics, sports and fitness, and the pursuit of optimal living.

Kathy and Victor exude devotion to the love of family. With four successful children who all attended Division I colleges as student athletes, they have always found that their greatest reward is gathering inspiration from each other.

NOTES

Prologue

Ponzio-Mouttaki, Amanda. The 22 Essentials of Marrakech Restaurants, January 7, 2020. Eater.com. A street vendor sells flatbreads, He, Gary. https://www.eater.com/maps/best-restaurants-marrakech-morocco

Chapter 1

Cascone, Sarah, ArtNet. Art World. Preserving the Sistine Chapel Is a Never-Ending Task. Art qqWorld. Artnet. March 28, 2019. "Preventative conservation" is the key to keeping the ceiling looking fresh. Art World. Artnet. March 28, 2019.

Fulford, Robert, column about art restoration in Italy. Globe and Mail, February 11, 1998.

Journal of Ancient Civilizations, The Journal of Ancient Civilizations (JAC) is published by the Institute for the History of Ancient Civilizations (IHAC), Northeast Normal University, Changchun. Due to his 30th anniversary in 2014 we publish the content list of vols. 1–28 (1986–2013) of JAC.

Chapter 2

Klainerman, S., Stability of Minkowski Space. In Encyclopedia of Mathematical Physics, 2006.

Mark, Joshua J. "Ancient Greece." Ancient History Encyclopedia. Last modified November 13, 2013.

Maura Ellyn; Maura McGinnis (2004). Greece: A Primary Source Cultural Guide. The Rosen Publishing Group. p. 8.

Kakissis, Joanna. Summit of the gods. The Greeks put gods on Olympus and men aspire to the same beautiful perspective. The Boston Globe. July 17, 2005.

United Nations Education, Scientific and Cultural Organization. World Heritage Convention. The Broader Region of Mount Olympus.

Jones, Gabriel H. "Pythia." Ancient History Encyclopedia. Published August 30, 2013.

United Nations Education, Scientific and Cultural Organization. World Heritage Convention. Archeological Site of Delphi.

United Nations Education, Scientific and Cultural Organization. World Heritage Convention. Archeological Site of Delphi.

National Library of Medicine. PubMed.

Bender DA (2003). Nutritional Biochemistry of the Vitamins. Cambridge University Press. p. 203. ISBN 978-1-139-43773-8. Archived from the original on 30 December 2016.

World Health Organization (2009). Stuart MC, Kouimtzi M, Hill SR (eds.). WHO Model Formulary 2008. World Health Organization. pp. 496, 500. hdl:10665/44053. ISBN 9789241547659.

Törnroth-Horsefield, S.; Neutze, R. (December 2008). "Opening and closing the metabolite gate". Proc. Natl. Acad. Sci. USA. 105 (50): 19565–19566.

US National Library of Medicine. National Institutes of Health.

Medically reviewed by Seunggu Han, M.D. - Written by Jill Seladi-Schuman, Ph.D. - Updated on March 21. 2018.

Middlemas, David, in xPharm: The Comprehensive Pharmacology Reference, 2007.

Chapter 3

Understanding Early Civilizations: A Comparative Study, Trigger, Bruce G., Cambridge University Press, 2007.

Maya, History.com Editors. A7&E Television Networks, October 29, 2009.

Davíd Carrasco. "Mesoamerica: An Overview". In Davíd Carrasco (ed). The Oxford Encyclopedia of Mesoamerican Cultures. Vol 2. New York: Oxford University Press, 2001. Pp 212 - 216 ISBN 9780195108156.

Otieno, Mark Owuor, World Atlas, January 31, 2018.

Burns, Robert, Auld Lang Syne. Scottish Poem written in 1788.

Chapter 4

Cunningham, Alexander (1875). *Archaeological Survey of India, Report for the Year 1872–1873, Vol. 5*. Calcutta: The Superintendent of Government. Archaeological Survey of India.

Parpola, Asko (19 May 2005). "Study of the Indus Script" (PDF). Archived from the original (PDF) on 6 March 2006. (50th ICES Tokyo Session).

Chapter 5

Sang-Hun, Choe (2016-09-26). "For South Koreans, a Long Detour to Their Holy Mountain". The New York Times. ISSN 0362-4331. Retrieved 2019-06-06.

Marder, Eve (4 October 2012). "Neuromodulation of Neuronal Circuits: Back to the Future". Neuron. 76 (1): 1–11.

doi:10.1016/j.neuron.2012.09.010. ISSN 0896-6273. PMC 3482119. PMID 23040802

Chapter 6

Peck, Douglas T. "Misconceptions and Myths Related to the Fountain of Youth and Juan Ponce de Leon's 1513 Exploration Voyage"(PDF). New World Explorers, Inc. Archived from the original (PDF)on 2008-04-09. Retrieved 2008-04-03.

Zorea, Aharon (2017). Finding the Fountain of Youth: The Science and Controversy Behind Extending Life and Cheating Death. Westport, CT: Greenwood Press. pp. 35–39. ISBN 978-1440837982.

Mandeville, John. The Travels of Sir John Mandeville. Accessed 24 Sept 2011.

Epidemiology Of Water Magnesium; Evidence of Contributions to Health Mildred S. Seelig, M.D., M.P.H., Master of American College of Nutrition; Adjunct Professor of Nutrition, School of Public Health, University of North Carolina, Chapel Hill (in Press: Proceedings of Mg Symposium, Vichy, France 2000)

Drye, William, Fountain of Youth, A mythical fountain capable of preserving life has been a popular legend for centuries.

Chapter 7

Ancient History Encyclopedia. The Ancient Mesopotamia Civilization. Mark, Joshua, J. March 14, 2018.

Kiger, Patrick J., How Mesopotamia became the Cradle of Civilization. November 10, 2020.

Mesopotamia, History.com Editors, Updated: September 30, 2019 - Original: November 30, 2017.

Mark, Joshua J., Ancient History Encyclopedia, March 14, 2018.

Neolithic Revolution, History.com, Updated: August 23, 2019, Original: January 12, 2018.

Chapter 8

The Geography of India: Sacred and Historic Places. The Rosen Publishing Group, Inc. 2010. p. 174. ISBN 978-1-61530-142-3. Retrieved 11 August 2020.

District Census Handbook – Bhopal" (PDF). Census of India. p. 35. Archived (PDF) from the original on 7 August 2015. Retrieved 22 September 2015.

John Falconer, James Waterhouse (2009). The Waterhouse albums: central Indian provinces. Mapin. ISBN 978-81-89995-30-0.

Whipps, Heather, Survival Dance: How Humans Waltzed Through the Ice Age. March 10, 2006.

Bachner-Melman R, Dina C, Zohar AH, Constantini N, Lerer E, Hoch S, et al. (2005) AVPR1a and SLC6A4 Gene Polymorphisms Are Associated with Creative Dance Performance. PLoS Genet 1(3): e42. https://doi.org/10.1371/journal.pgen.0010042

Bhimbetka rock shelters, Madhya Pradesh, India.

Peter N. Peregrine; Melvin Ember (2003). *Encyclopedia of Prehistory: Volume 8: South and Southwest Asia*. Springer Science. pp. 315–317. ISBN 978-0-306-46262-7.

Chapter 9

Soar Above One of the Most Awe-Inspiring Waterfalls on Earth". National Geographic. 19 March 2019. Retrieved 9 June 2020.

"Victoria Falls". World Digital Library. 1890–1925. Retrieved 1 June 2013.

Scheffel, Richard L.; Wernet, Susan J., eds. (1980). Natural Wonders of the World. United States of America: Reader's Digest Association, Inc. pp. 402–403. ISBN 0-89577-087-3.

"Definitions [of love]" (PDF). mbcarlington.com. Greek word study on Love. Archived from the original (PDF) on 2014-11-27.

Shiel, William C., MD, FACP, FACR. Medical Author. Medical Definition of Oxytocin.

Shiel, William C., MD, FACP, FACR. Medical Author. Medical Definition of Serotonin.

Shiel, William C., MD, FACP, FACR. Medical Author. Medical Definition of Dopamine.

Shiel, William C., MD, FACP, FACR. Medical Author. Medical Definition of Endorphins.

Roman, Kaia. "The Brain Chemicals That Make You Happy (And How to Trigger Them)." Brain Renewal. 2021. Retrieved 26 February 2021.

A free ebook edition is available with the purchase of this book.

To claim your free ebook edition:

Visit MorganJamesBOGO.com
Sign your name CLEARLY in the space
Complete the form and submit a photo of
the entire copyright page
You or your friend can download the ebook
to your preferred device

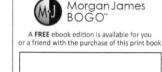
Print & Digital Together Forever.

Snap a photo

Free ebook

Read anywhere

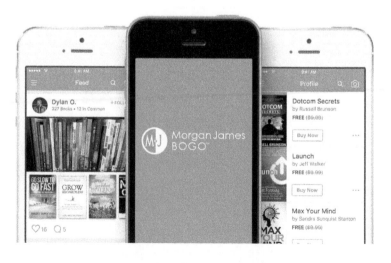

9 781631 953699